The Yoni Egg

"I applaud Lilou Macé's fantastic contribution to the wellness of womb wisdom around the world. It is glorious to see these feminine mysteries out there for all to find. Gift all those women you love with this book and they will be truly thankful."

ANAIYA SOPHIA,
AUTHOR OF *FIERCE FEMININE RISING*
AND *SACRED SEXUAL UNION*

The Yoni Egg

Reveal and Release
the Sacred Feminine Within

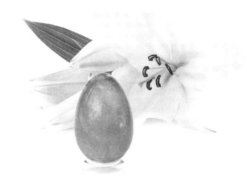

Lilou Macé

Translated by Jon E. Graham

Destiny Books
Rochester, Vermont

Destiny Books
One Park Street
Rochester, Vermont 05767
www.DestinyBooks.com

Destiny Books is a division of Inner Traditions International

Originally published in French under the title *L'Oeuf de Yoni: le féminin révélé et libéré* by Leduc.s Éditions (a division of Eddison Books Ltd./Editions Leduc) 29 boulevard Raspail, 75007 Paris, France.

Note to the reader: This book is intended as an informational guide. The remedies, approaches, and techniques described herein are meant to supplement, and not to be a substitute for, professional medical care or treatment. They should not be used to treat a serious ailment without prior consultation with a qualified health care professional.

Cataloging-in-Publication Data for this title is available from the Library of Congress

ISBN 978-1-62055-865-2 (print)
ISBN 978-1-62055-866-9 (ebook)

Printed and bound in the United States by Versa Press, Inc.

10 9 8 7 6 5 4 3 2 1

Text design and layout by Virginia Scott Bowman
This book was typeset in Garamond Premier Pro, Gill Sans, and Avenir with
    Gotham Pro used as the display typeface
Color photos of the yoni eggs by Muriel Despiau

To send correspondence to the author of this book, mail a first-class letter to the author c/o Inner Traditions • Bear & Company, One Park Street, Rochester, VT 05767, and we will forward the communication, or contact the author directly at **www.liloumace.com/en.**

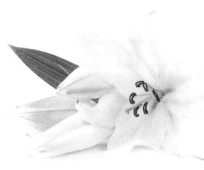

Contents

PART ONE
· · · · · · · · · · · · · ·

Discovering the Secrets of Your Yoni

PART TWO
· · · · · · · · · · · · · ·

How to Choose the Perfect Yoni Egg for You

A Note about
the Yoni Egg Practices

The information presented in this book is based on the author's personal experience, knowledge, and research on women and the effects of the yoni egg. The yoni egg, or jade egg, has been used for a variety of purposes for thousands of years, dating back to the empresses and concubines of ancient China. The practices described in this book are not a substitute for professional medical treatment or an invitation to throw caution to the wind. If you are suffering from a mental, emotional, or physical disorder, you are advised to consult with your health practitioner or therapist before beginning practices using the yoni egg. This book does not claim to provide medical diagnoses or prescriptions for illnesses, pains, disorders, or any other physical conditions. We cannot be held responsible for the consequences of this practice or the poor use of the information provided by this book. If you perform certain exercises without following the instructions, commentary, and warnings, you will be solely responsible for your practice.

Foreword

By Mantak Chia

The emperors of ancient China maintained harems filled with women responsible for attending to their pleasures. One of the essential skills for these women involved the practice and mastery of the jade egg.

The woman was expected to insert the jade egg into her vagina and practice with it. When the time came, she was given a test. A gold wire was attached to the egg. The other end of the wire was then attached to a heavy throne. The woman would use her vaginal muscles to pull on the gold wire until it broke, thereby demonstrating the strength of her vagina.

At this stage of mastery, the concubine was strong enough to squeeze the emperor's penis at will when it was inside her vagina. She did this not only to procure greater pleasure for the ruler but also to prevent the emperor from passing beyond his "point of no return." With no emission of sperm, pregnancy was avoided.

I learned this from my Taoist teacher. He also gave me detailed instructions on how to use this ancient imperial practice for the health and pleasure of both women and men. Now, having observed the positive reactions of my students over the years, I am happy to learn that Lilou is passing these valuable teachings on to a much larger audience. Those lucky women who dare to experiment and achieve the wonders offered by the yoni egg practice will appreciate the gift of this vital information, with its emphasis on good health and good chi.

MANTAK CHIA, a student of several Taoist masters, founded the Healing Tao System in North America in 1979 and developed it worldwide as European Tao Yoga and Universal Healing Tao. He has taught and certified tens of thousands of students and instructors from all over the world and tours the United States annually, giving workshops and lectures. He is the director of the Tao Garden Health Spa and the Universal Healing Tao training center in northern Thailand and is the author of more than fifty books, including *Taoist Foreplay, Inner Smile, Cosmic Fusion, Sexual Reflexology,* and the bestselling *The Multi-Orgasmic Man.*

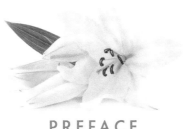

In Complete Privacy

I first heard about yoni eggs in Chiang Mai, Thailand, several years ago. I was there to interview Mantak Chia about longevity and Taoist pratices, when I discovered that practice. I was immediately intrigued by this small, oval, polished stone and wanted to know more. I wanted to learn more about it and test it. I was excited to discover a "women's secret" that would allow me to free my female energy, reveal my inner beauty, and restore my self-confidence. I was single, and those concepts became a recurring theme for me.

I cannot say that, at the beginning, I felt completely casual about inserting the egg into my body. It quickly made me aware of a few things, mainly my ignorance about my intimate anatomy. It became clear that I was more interested in this part of my body as an object of desire, pleasure, and lust than as something that could reveal the power of my inner femininity. I was confronted by my shame, my carelessness, and my ignorance, but thanks to this small object, I was immediately prepared to learn more about the yoni.

The yoni? No, *my* yoni! What a sweet name for describing this most intimate part of my body! What tenderness and complicity is given off by this word for describing my sex organ! I placed my right hand over this part of my body and, while my heart beat wildly, said, "My yoni," in a tone of friendliness and goodwill, and I felt the first signs of a gentle complicity and an enthralling chapter of my life.

What could truly be hidden in this secret cave? Could my yoni conceal secrets even more extraordinary than pleasure and enjoyment?

Several days later, after having asked a few questions about this mysterious yoni egg, I decided to make my first attempt. "Oooohhhh!" "Oops!" "Aaahhhhh!" And finally "gotcha!" as my egg was sucked in by my yoni! The stone was now peacefully and serenely positioned inside me. I took a deep breath and stood up. I could not feel it inside me, yet *something was different.*

Over the following days, I quickly noticed that my relationship to men was evolving. I felt more trusting, calm, and sensual. I had less and less need for attention, compliments, and love. I had rediscovered this part of my body; I was giving it my attention and listening to it more every day. The more my sex organ relaxed and opened, the more at home in myself I felt. I began giving off a subtle, almost tangible power. Men became interested in me no longer just sexually but for the woman I was! This was a first. Could my perception, presence, and attention have transformed so quickly? Was it the effect of the stone, the aura released by my yoni, my quest, or simply my new questions that allowed me to experience these new events, or was it simply coincidence?

My regular experience with the yoni egg, accompanied by expert advice, quickly led me to realize that coincidence had nothing to do with it. With one full year of practice under my belt, I returned to Thailand to film a series of interviews that would allow me to become better informed about the amazing secrets of the yoni egg, and to make these secrets better known.

Broadcasted on YouTube, these interviews inspired thousands of women to experiment with the power of the yoni egg practice. Faced with growing demand from viewers who came my way, I began offering yoni eggs on my website (see the resources on page 165). This led to a tsunami of questions and inspiring testimonies. Just as the yoni egg had immediately impressed itself upon mc, the response from thousands of women made it immediately evident that I had to write this book. I felt a desire to share the liberating qualities of this practice and to bring this women's secret back into the world. It became obvious that I had to follow my soul and heart's calling into this grand adventure into the sacred feminine. I would be led.

This book will show you how you can use the yoni egg at all times in your life as a woman, but it will also teach you that you cannot just use it anyway you choose. Inserting an object into your body is, understandably, grounds for questioning. Some readers will be more at ease than others at first contact with the egg. The yoni egg practice is adaptable to many individuals of various ages, lifestyles, and experiences—including women who have had painful experiences—and also in accordance with our feelings and desires.

Like all practices, using the yoni egg requires regularity, listening to your inner self, and taking the time to experience the messages and changes within your body and in your life. I learned that it was an intuitive process and that giving a voice to our yoni was precious in our evolution into the sacred feminine.

In complete complicity and in complete respect of your yoni, this practice will allow understanding of your inner wisdom and magnificence within, and it will help you activate the true power that has not yet seen the light inside of you—the power of your radiant femininity.

Many women have admitted to me that they feel more alive, serene, and "sensual" thanks to their egg. It is my wish that the egg can help us to be confident and free in our body and in making decisions that truly matter to us. We have a voice that is calling to be heard. We are evolving as women to the next stage, to participate more actively and freely in a new world where old preoccupations such as intellect, competition, fear, and perfection are no longer the way to thrive and succeed.

This book is meant to be a practical guide to understanding many of the benefits offered by yoni eggs, choosing the size and gemstone of your own egg, and pursuing this practice with ease and freedom. To achieve all this, I asked the advice of health professionals and gemologists, who added their expertise to that of practitioners who are specialists in the yoni egg exercises and the sacred feminine. You'll find all of these wonderful contributors speaking in their own words throughout this book; most of the advice and information recorded here comes from the interviews that I conducted. (You can view the full interviews online on YouTube; see page 167 for the interview link titles.) You will also find here testimonies from women of all ages and all walks of life who wish to share their personal experiences and advice about yoni eggs with their sisters.

I cannot claim that I've gathered here all the information existing on this subject, but I hope I've managed to integrate the essence of the information necessary to initiate yourself into the practice of the yoni egg with complete confidence. My intention is for the contents of this book to awaken in you a dimension that you may never have known before. It is my intention that, by freeing your body from restrictive memories, you will find the courage to realize and manifest your potent inner beauty in complete serenity. I also wish for you to become witness to a new world hatching before your very eyes, sparkling with excitement and joy.

I am wholeheartedly with you in this new stage of your life.

—Lilou Macé

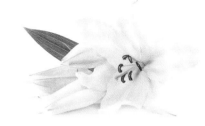

Acknowledgments

I would like to thank the entire crew of my French publisher, Éditions Leduc, with whom I first published this book, and particularly my editor, Liza, who believed in my book and the importance of its contents. Thank you for putting everything together to make this book what it is. Thanks to all the men and all the women who shared—from near or far—in the challenges and joys of the editing and production, without whom this book would not exist. You are all the best!

Thanks to Mantak Chia, who brought the jade egg to the West so many years ago and has written such important books about men, women, and Tao and who created the Tao Garden Health Spa and Resort in Thailand. I first discovered the jade eggs there, and I love recharging my batteries in this place that offers so many innovative yet ancient massages and techniques. Each time I go there it opens to me new possibilities for expansion and relaxation. I would also like to thank him for his interviews and for having passed on his wisdom and knowledge to so many wonderful instructors of Tao across the world. He is a guide for many. I would like to particularly thank Sarina, José, Aisha, Jutta, Shashi, Solla, and Minke for having generously shared their knowledge in all the interviews they granted me.

Thanks also to all the yoni egg users who agreed to respond to my questions and allowed me to share their testimonies in the pages of this book. Your contribution is immense, both for the creation of this book and for the thousands of women who will read it. Sharing our secrets and fears, woman to woman, in such an authentic way is priceless.

My infinite thanks to you, my dear co-creators. You know who you are. You have watched my interviews online, shared them, opened yourself to new possibilities, and inspired countless people around you by creating lasting results. Bravo! You are my rock.

The intention behind this book is so large and so beautiful that I could not do it on my own. Many people have participated in its creation from beginning to end. I would, however, like to thank all those who were not a part of this project for very long but still contributed, despite everything, to its beauty and success.

I would especially like to thank Marie-Pierre, Séverine, Corinne, François, Dimitri, Muriel, Laura, Fabrice, Arnaud, Caroline, Stéphane, Mariette, Lara, Elizabeth, Phi-Haï Phan, and the Inner Traditions team that made this book available in the United States, a country dear to my heart where I first started interviewing.

I want to thank my fiancé and partner, Mickaël, who gave me his unconditional support every day to live my life's mission fully—without you, my life would not be the same. Thank you for helping me discover what is love and what is not. Thank you for your openness, joy, enthusiasm, sense of organization, energy, and heart. I love you. You are my angel, my guardian, and my knight.

And finally, I want to thank all women reading this book, passing it along, sharing the secrets of the yoni egg with others. What I have seen happening in France with this practice is nothing but a miracle. We can trust our body. No media or authority can tell us what is best for us as we are claiming our wisdom in this new era. Well done, sisters!

PART ONE

· · · · · · · · · · · · · · · ·

*Discovering
the Secrets of
Your Yoni*

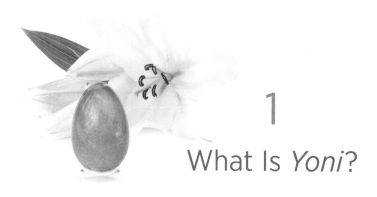

1
What Is *Yoni*?

Everyone has their own little name for the most intriguing and intimate part of our anatomy—in other words, our sexual organs. Our wide range of names, from the most poetic to the most vulgar, evolved with our society and with the evolution of woman.

I was taking part in a tantra workshop when I first encountered the term *yoni* and immediately fell under its spell. *Yoni.* Gentle, delicate, exotic . . . it was as if I had been transported to a new paradigm to explore new possibilities. At last, I had a gracious, mysterious, and respectful name to describe this part of my body.

After some research, I discovered that the term *yoni* (which comes from Sanskrit, the ancestral Indo-European language) describes much more than the outer part of my sex organs. Physically speaking, *yoni* designates not only the outside (the mons pubis or pubic mound, urethral opening, lips, and clitoris) but also the inside (including the uterus, vagina, pelvic floor, ovaries, and fallopian tubes) of the female sex organ. It is fantastic to finally have a name to define the entirety of this part of my body.

Universally speaking, the yoni is the seat of our creative force and our female energy; it is the temple of an inner wisdom. By liberating certain memories, traumas, and energies stored in this part of our body, we can gain access to an unprecedented blossoming and revelations.

The yoni is therefore not just another body part. It is the foundation of an ancient yet modern approach to woman's sexuality that opens onto a much broader knowledge of the sacred feminine.

"It is an extraordinary space. The more you are able to explore it, the more doors you will open, and then more doors opening to the inside, and this gives you access to the immensity of life," explains Aisha Sieburth, author and advanced instructor of Tao (certified by Mantak Chia).

The good news is that this knowledge has never been truly lost. It goes on as it has since the dawn of time, ever present in our bodies as women. It is hidden within us like a treasure, inside a place we have forgotten to cultivate, to honor, and which we no longer remember how to connect in order to gain access to its true secrets.

The good news is that with practices and rituals we unlock its mysteries and free ourselves from ages of patriarchy! As I see it, intimate knowledge of our yoni allows us to resolve part of the paradox that we live as women: *We are carrying inside that which we so desperately seek on the outside. A profound journey inside ourselves will guide us toward a radiant era where women are really seen for who they are.*

With this book, I offer a way for women to explore the secrets of our yoni, like a key that lets you enter a realm in which you will unleash and reveal to yourself and the world the power and the beauty within.

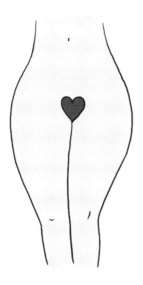

Figure 1.1. The yoni, the heart of the sacred feminine within

A QUICK LESSON IN ANATOMY

In case you skipped your health classes, here is a brief summary that will be important to keep in mind for getting the most out of the practices described in this book.

When we explore the outside areas of our yoni, the first thing we see is the mons pubis, also known as the mons veneris (meaning mound of Venus). This rounded layer of tissue is located in the center and lowest part of our belly. Starting in puberty, it manifests one of the main secondary characteristics of our sexual nature: pubic hair, which can be more or less luxurious. Everyone has their own "yoni fashion." . . . But let's move on and get back to anatomy!

The mons veneris has a downward-pointing triangular shape. At the bottom point appears the clitoris, at the juncture of the two large lips, or labia. These outer lips conceal smaller inner lips that are thinner in texture and more sensitive; they grow larger when we are aroused.

Below this area we find three orifices: the one that releases urine (the urethral opening), the vagina, and the anus. The vagina is a canal that leads to the G-spot and the uterus.

Understanding and Knowing Your Yoni Thanks to Your Egg

Introducing an object like a stone egg into the vagina is not an obvious and natural thing to do. Many women are nervous that, once inserted, the egg will remain stuck inside them or escape into the depths of their bodies.

To help you get past this fear, think of your vagina as a room. It has walls and a "ceiling." The egg will not be able to go anywhere.

❝ *In the beginning, I was scared by the size of my egg, and of losing it inside my yoni . . .*

ALEXANDRA ❞

Once you have overcome these initial anatomical fears, you will be free to undertake some real inner work on much deeper fears waiting to be released.

    ❝ *I had a lot of worries. If it was too big or heavy, would it stay inside of me? What if I kept it inside too long; would it get stuck in my yoni for several months? Finally, when the time came, everything went just fine!*

    — MARIE ❞

Aisha Sieburth offers this reassurance: "This part of our body is often somewhat overlooked and somewhat hidden, if not, more accurately, unknown. Using a yoni egg is about learning our anatomy and knowing it intimately."

For those who are afraid that the yoni egg will somehow disappear inside them, a little lesson of anatomy should prove helpful.

Our yoni consists of several organs and muscles, all connected to each other inside a cavity: the pelvic cavity. This area is entered through the vulva, which is all the external genital organs of the woman. The vulva consists of the mons veneris, the vaginal vestibule, the labia majora and the labia minora (the large and small lips), the clitoris, the corpus cavernosum, the vestibular bulbs, and the vestibular glands. The labia minora lead directly into the vagina, which is the channel connecting the vulva to the cervix.

Here we find the perineum, the area between the pubic symphysis (an ungainly name describing the joint between the right and left pubic bones, at the midline of the pelvis) and the sacrum and coccyx. The perineal muscles permit to hold of all the external genital organs, which is why it is so important to have a well-toned perineum. (We will explore your own perineal tone in the next chapter.)

The vagina, therefore, leads to the cervix, which is the terminal part of the uterus. The uterus, a cone-shaped muscular organ, consists of three layers of smooth muscles that allow it to contract. The interior of the uterus is covered by an extremely vascular mucous membrane,

Insertion of the egg

Spinal column

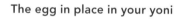

Ovary

Uterus

Yoni Egg

Vagina

Rectum

The egg in place in your yoni

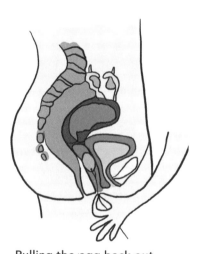

**Pulling the egg back out
of the yoni**

Figure 1.2. The egg's placement inside the yoni

the famous endometrium, which grows thicker each month during the menstrual cycle. If pregnancy does not occur, the endometrium destroys this additional growth under the influence of certain sexual hormones, thereby causing menstruation. Our uterus, which is connected by more or less taut membranes, dances, sways, and remains flexible. This enables it to find its proper place in the body and to enjoy maximum functionality.

Beginning to have a clearer vision of our female anatomy is the very first benefit from the yoni egg practice. Our yoni should be a soft, warm, and welcoming space.

> **❝** *Thanks to the egg, I discovered the texture of my vagina as well as its heat.... When I took the egg back out, I had a deep emotional reaction when I realized how warm it was.*
> ANNE **❞**

The Feminine Fluids

There is another important topic to cover in this explanation: our three feminine fluids! The first fluid appears during arousal to lubricate the vagina. The second fluid is emitted at the moment of orgasm. The third, which is experienced naturally by what Jacques Salomé* calls "spring women" or "fountain women," is available to most of us through practice. This third fluid that we as women can "ejaculate" abundantly from our yoni is misunderstood and much research is being undertaken about this phenomenon. Many women who have experienced it say it gives a feeling of freeing themselves from past emotions and memories. It gives them an amazing experience of lasting waves of pleasure and serenity.

I once had a session with José Toirán, who was trained by Mantak Chia. This practitioner is special and unique. He has the ability to help women experience female ejaculation. I was skeptical at first, but since I was single at the time and visiting the Tao Garden in Thailand, I felt

---

*Jacques Salomé is a French psychosociologist and author of the book *L'effet source* [The spring effect], which investigates the phenomenon of "spring women"—that is, women who are able to ejaculate. —Ed.

open to such an unusual and extraordinary experience. I can testify that it was a unique and life-changing experience for me. I did not know that my body was capable of it and that I could experience so much peaceful-ness. It was not sexual. It was a sacred experience, freeing me from many memories. I am now fully conscious that the knowledge stored in our bodies, released during our orgasms and liberated via our fluids, is still a big mystery to most of us and that we are a long way from exploring it openly. I am grateful that I listened and acted upon my intuition. I was ready. I am so grateful that I had the courage to experience it.

I am nervous and my body is shivering despite the warm weather in Thailand. I am naked beneath some white bath towels, and José is massaging my body with coconut oil. He teaches me to breathe in unison with him and to suck his fingers with my yoni (he is wearing latex gloves) and then push them out with my uterus. Under his guidance, my breathing is shifting until we are breathing as one. It is as if I am making love to myself, as if I am offering this gift to myself. My sex opens, the rhythms increase in intensity, and I come. The spring opens and water flows out of me in abundance. I feel majestic. I feel like a goddess. I am forever transformed.*

José believes that all women are capable of ejaculating and that it is healing. He has a technique that he teaches during his sessions. He has also begun studies with a team of scientists to explain this phenomenon in women, which he hopes to make more visible and better accepted.

Now that we can see a bit more clearly on the subject of the yoni, let's study the activities that can help us activate all the energy that is slum-bering inside it and see how we can free our essential femininity and restore our confidence in ourselves.

---

*This is an extract from my book *Je suis célibataire et ça me plait* [I am single and I like it] (Paris: Éditions Trédaniel, 2016).

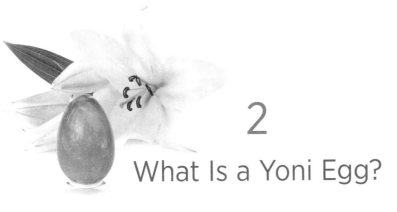

2
What Is a Yoni Egg?

"Women carry everything inside them. They do not have anything on the outside to train with. It is easier for men because everything is on the outside. They can touch and pull on it, as opposed to women, who need a tool to do that," says Jutta Kellenberger, an expert on women's issues, Taoism, meditation, and yoni eggs.

The yoni egg is an object made from a semiprecious or precious stone that is intended to be placed in our yoni. It is historically called a jade egg, as imperial jade was traditionally used to craft the earliest eggs. It may also be referred to as an energetic egg.

The egg provides many benefits for our well-being, vitality, and sexuality, which I will describe in detail in this chapter. One of the most well-known benefits is how it strengthens the pelvic floor through the vaginal channel.

When you work out or play a sport, you do not expect to obtain significant results without exercising regularly and working your muscles even just minimally. Well, the same is true for yoni eggs. As they come in a variety of sizes, they will give your yoni something to work with! Your vaginal channel will then become a tool for strengthening your pelvic floor. The pelvic floor is made up of a series of muscles in the shape of a hammock that hangs between the front and back of the body, and it provides support to a number of important organs.

By following the practices and exercises explained in this book, you will be able to improve the tone of your pelvic floor and more. And that's not all. The yoni egg has an equally important impact on our self-confidence, bringing consciousness to this part of our body, helping to reconnect to our inner wisdom and power, our sexuality, our vitality. But most of all it helps support us in being free to be who we really are: goddesses. Women's personal motivations for using the egg have evolved since the days it was first used in ancient China, and they will vary in accordance with the individual's age, needs, and desires.

"The yoni egg is like a jewel or treasure with which you weave a friendship. It allows you to form a bond with this part of our body that you can then explore and discover," Aisha Sieburth teaches us.

Yoni eggs are carved and sculpted from a wide variety of stones. Each kind of stone has unique lithotherapeutic properties; which stone an individual chooses for her yoni egg will thus depend on her needs, intuition, and desires. In chapter 5 we will examine the various sizes and kinds of stones that can be used for a yoni egg, listed in accordance with their specific benefits.

The eggs are polished until they shine and possess varying degrees of transparency, depending on what kind of stone they birthed from. They all come in three sizes, the use of which will depend on your body, age, and level of experience with the egg.

As Aisha Sieburth points out, "The yoni egg possesses a mineral substance that comes out of the earth, a very noble substance that we will use to awaken the sacred cauldron of our femininity, that space that gives birth to creative energies."

All this might seem extremely mysterious to you at this stage; trust me, you shall be initiated into all the egg's secrets as you read through this book.

The practice of the yoni egg goes back to the dawn of time in China and has now been adapted to the active, modern women we are today.

THE LEGENDARY ORIGINS OF THE EGG

Mantak Chia was the first Taoist master to talk about the jade egg in his books (in the 1970s). The many instructors and experts whom I interviewed to learn more about this practice, such as Aisha Sieburth, Jutta Kellenberger, Sarina Stone, Minke de Vos, Shashi Solluna, and José Toirán, were all trained by this pioneering figure.

"In ancient times, this technique was reserved for the queen, the princess, and the concubines. Female Taoist instructors would come to teach them the 'art of love making,'" Mantak Chia told me in a captivating intimate interview I had with him at his home in Chiang Mai, Thailand.

The history of the jade egg, or yoni egg, therefore goes back more than two thousand years in ancient China. At the request of the emperor, the empress and hundreds of concubines were initiated, in the greatest secrecy, into the practice of the egg so that they could strengthen the power of their sexual organ and preserve their youth and vitality, ensuring that they would be able to make love divinely well with the emperor!

Controlling the contractions of their vagina allowed them to control the emperor's excitement, which ensured that the energy generated by lovemaking would rise to his higher centers. Filled with universal and cosmic energy, the emperor could then connect with a wiser and greater dimension of his self and thus be in a position to make the best decisions for his kingdom.

Although the primary objective of this practice was the emperor's pleasure (and the mastery of his ejaculations), the more skill and dexterity his sexual partners gained in this art, the greater their potency and power would become. His favorites were those who had become experts in this domain.

THE YONI EGG AND THE MODERN WOMAN

Yoni egg practice has clearly evolved with our evolution. We are no longer under any obligation to give all our powers to the emperor. Instead, we use these practices to empower ourselves.

The yoni egg is readily adaptable to the daily realities a woman deals with today: work, family, aspirations, obligations, loss of bearings, the search for greater meaning, and so on, along with all the stress these factors can create in our daily lives. It allows a woman to reveal herself, unleash her power as she follows the path of inner transformations that the yoni egg encourages her to go for. "The jade egg is a tool that can give us concrete aid for putting this process in motion," Aisha Sieburth tells us, adding:

The practice of the egg was conceived for awakening the sacred dimension of female energy, and for reconnecting to its divinity, its healing energy, and its inner peaceful strength so that we might rediscover autonomy and balance in the health of our bodies, hearts, spirituality, and minds, while connecting to greater universal forces.

Because of the way it is shaped, the egg will become one with the yoni. Regular use of the egg, combined with periods of rest and observation, will allow us to know ourselves better, awaken our creative and sexual energies, and also feel intuitively guided when making decisions. The practice is interspersed with numerous exercises, which will evolve over time.

Mirroring the evolution of the women in society, the yoni egg practice has also adapted to our modern needs and desires, thereby allowing us to birth ourselves into a new era, without past conditionings, free to shine our light. I will therefore share with you simple yet powerful rituals to connect with the sacred feminine in the last chapter of this book.

WHAT ABOUT GEISHA OR BEN WA BALLS?

Often viewed as a pleasure device, a means of giving the vagina an iron constitution, or a sex toy, geisha balls (also known as ben wa balls, orgasm balls, or Venus balls), contrary to yoni eggs, are used most often in pairs (they are sold in packs of two).

Advanced Practice

In more advanced yoni egg practice, women can also use two eggs. José Toirán explained to me that when women use two small yoni eggs, we can practice moving them around inside, separating and bringing them back together to master the various muscle rings of our vagina, thereby allowing us to attain greater control of our bodies and pleasures.

What are geisha balls made from? They are often made of silicone or plastic and more rarely from steel, glass, or even stone. Their movement is triggered by movement of the woman's body, and, like yoni eggs, the balls build the various muscles that form the pelvic floor and strengthen the perineum. They also create vibrations and therefore cause a kind of pleasurable sensation when they are carried.

They are different from yoni eggs in shape (they are round), size, and weight, and they are more often just inserted in the yoni rather than used in any kind of practice. A yoni egg, on the other hand, is generally pierced and is used in a number of evolutionary practices, which vary in accordance with the egg's weight and size. The possibility of increasing the weight, varying the practices, and being more creative in its use offers a great number of benefits than what can be guaranteed by geisha balls.

❝ *A friend of mine was using geisha balls made of plastic for physiotherapy. I also bought some. But I did not like what they were made of. I can 'wear' an egg all morning without any problem.*
CATHERINE ❞

Geisha balls make it possible to work on local areas through contraction. But here is the thing: we cannot expect to obtain better yoni tone by only contracting and relaxing the muscles. Furthermore, the balls are often too light or too small for effective muscle work. Most importantly, it is not possible to attach weights to them to get a real workout. In fact, the muscle responsible for the tone of the pelvic floor is not even inside our vaginal channel, which makes the Kegel exercises that have been adapted for use with geisha balls almost useless. Moreover, Dr. Arnold Kegel, who created these exercises, advised that they be practiced with weights to increase the resistance.

THE SYMBOLISM OF THE EGG

Holding a yoni egg in your hand for the first time is both intimidating and exciting. Though it seems like a small, round shiny object, it has visceral power; you can feel it. The egg is a symbol of life, fertility, rebirth, and a new start. It can also evoke tenderness, happiness, the inner child, and intrauterine life.*

On the symbolic level, the egg can strongly embody the woman and her personal expectations, which will vary radically from one individual to the next.

> " This egg truly liberated my femininity and sexuality. Its symbol freed me from childbirth and allowed me to mentally welcome a being into my belly when I had been someone who experienced difficulties concerning motherhood and bringing a child into the world.
>
> HÉLÈNE "

The egg also represents unity, the reunion of yin and yang, the areas of light and shadow that coexist in each of us. It is a material expression of fertility and birth, as well as the union of male and female. It is the source, the origin, and the starting point. It contains and protects. Wearing a yoni egg gives many women the sensation of being one with it and of finding their true place. It can be seen as a seed of conscious light that we carry inside of ourselves; one that will grow with time, observations, practices, and actions aligned with our true heart's desires.

---

*Intrauterine life is defined as the period of existence between conception and birth. —Ed.

The yoni egg is an evolutionary tool to support our growth and the big changes and challenges we are currently facing.

> ❝ *I discovered a new sensation of wholeness when I wore the egg.*
>
> Sᴏᴘʜɪᴇ ❞

For Aisha Sieburth, who teaches the practice of the jade egg in her workshops and trainings, the egg is the symbol of the work we are all called on to do: inner work, rather than outer work, to reconnect to a deeper place and open the many doors to the ancestral knowledge for which we are the guardians. "The inner work that is required here allows the unification of the whole. We become like an egg in turn," she says.

The yoni egg is also a symbol of the creative energy that we carry inside, as well as the liberation of our *chi* (or *ki*), vital energy that can become imprisoned in certain parts of the body, such as the yoni, in response to trauma. Working with the egg, as we shall see later, consists of massaging the yoni to free energy.

Jutta Kellenberger confirms this.

I often call it the "energetic egg" instead of the "jade egg" because it gives us a lot of energy. When someone does the exercises to strengthen the pelvic muscles, she feels totally energized, totally galvanized! It gives us so much life! So much energy stuck in this spot will be freed with time and practice!

REFLEXOLOGY AND THE YONI EGG

You have very likely heard of acupuncture, foot reflexology, or shiatsu massage. These Eastern healing techniques are based on the circulation of energy through channels called meridians that run throughout the body. Stimulation of specific points along these meridians can improve energy flow, relieve energy congestion, and activate related organs and physiological systems. Depending on the case, the practitioner will insert a needle into these points, sometimes called acupoints or reflexology points, or massage them to encourage energy circulation.

The meridians, each with its own trajectory, cross through all the organs of the body, including the vagina. Thus, as Jutta Kellenberger explains, "when we are exercising with the egg, we activate all the meridians and organs of our body."

According to traditional Chinese medicine (TCM), reflexology points make it possible to stimulate the energy of this or that organ, or to work on energy that has become congested so that it can be freed and start circulating again. For example, a meridian at the entrance of the vagina connects it to the bladder and kidneys (see figure 2.1). The center of the vagnia has a connection to the liver and spleen. Climbing higher, we find the lungs and, just below the cervix, the heart. The arrangement is exactly the same for men. The head of the penis is connected to the heart, and so on. Mantak Chia has explained sexual reflexology in a number of his books.

We have begun to get a glimpse of the entire energetic dimension of the yoni and sacred sexuality. Minke de Vos, an experienced Taoist instructor, sheds new light on this point for us.

> *The kidneys are at the opening of the yoni, right at the bottom; it is like a miniature human being. The liver and the spleen are in the middle of the yoni, and above them, toward the cervix, are the heart and lungs. The deeper the yoni is penetrated, the closer one comes to the heart. And if the heart opens, the energy will then rise through the core channel to the crown. You can open a core channel with your yoni and sacred sexuality and then bring all the chakras into alignment.*

In this way, working with a yoni egg will encourage the cleansing of the various regions of the yoni, our "jade palace," and allow for a rising circulation of energy.

Aisha Sieburth has no doubt about this whatsoever.

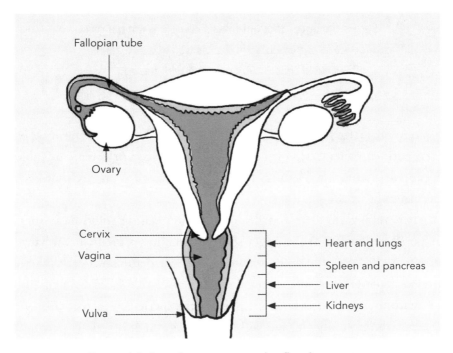

Figure 2.1. Female anatomy and reflexology points

We are going to be able to work with our emotions, with the elements of nature that have a connection with our organs. The elements of water, wood, earth, fire, metal, air, and so forth shall come see us inside the jade palace, located inside our body, to help us cleanse the wounds and old things, and by this leave room for our true nature.

TESTING THE TONE OF YOUR PERINEUM

Before beginning yoni egg energy work, and to ensure that the practice keeps its promises, let's take a moment to test the tone of your perineum. This will help you select the right size for your yoni egg and prepare for its insertion and use in your vagina.

" *Before the egg, I thought I was a complete wimp. I gained*
confidence in myself on a physical as well as a sexual level.
Because of that, I value my work with the egg.

CARINE "

Several factors can quickly tell you about the state of the tone of your perineum. To start with, if you are incontinent, or you are not able to stop urinating when you try to, then there is a good chance that your perineum lacks adequate tone.

It is important that you find a long and lasting solution as soon as possible, instead of finding a shortcut, such as a medicine. That is not enough. You need reeducation with a certified health care practitioner, depending on which stage you are at. After a certain age, due to anatomy, childbirth, and various other experiences, a reduction in tone is common, and it can cause some more or less serious personal health problems. At this point the yoni egg can help, but it is best used proactively.

Three Simple Tests of Perineal Tone

1. While urinating, after emptying more than half of your bladder, try to stop the stream of urine by squeezing your perineal muscles several times. If you can manage to stop the flow, your perineum is functioning normally. If the flow is reduced but not completely stopped, you have a loss of tone. If you are unable to alter the flow of urine at all, it is urgent that you begin to take care of your body and contact a health care practitioner who will evaluate and guide you in the first steps of your recovery. I will also explain some practices intended to restore tone to the perineum later in the book.

2. Wash your hands and then lie down on your bed. Squeeze your vagina as tightly as possible and try to insert your thumb into it. If you are able to insert your thumb, the tone of your perineum is good. If you are not able to insert your thumb, you might be too contracted, too tense. Exercising with small yoni eggs will help you

relax it. We will revisit this topic as this can apply to women who have experienced traumatic sexual situations in their past, forcing the yoni to shut down.

3. For more open-minded couples, ask your partner to help you by inserting a finger into your vagina. Squeeze your vagina as tightly as you can around the finger. Can your partner feel your inner strength? The stronger it feels, as if your partner's finger is being sucked in deeper, the better the tone of your perineum. The same holds true for your practice with the yoni egg, which will take up a position in the depths of your vagina. We will talk about this again.

If you have the slightest doubt, ask your gynecologist, midwife, or physical therapist to do a precise evaluation of your perineal tone. As you insert the yoni egg the first time, you will also get a clear evaluation of your yoni's strength!

3
Gaining Access to the Wonders of the Egg

The yoni egg practice offers many advantages for both women and men as well as individuals and couples. Its purpose is to allow you to better know your body and what you find pleasurable, as well as how to take care of yourself, gain confidence, release tension, restore a joyful state of personal health, and rebuild vitality and tone in your perineum.

Let's start by looking at what the egg provides on a daily basis for the majority of us.

THE POSITIVE EFFECTS ON YOUR DAILY FULFILLMENT AS A WOMAN

Provides Awareness and Kindness

Needing to take care of ourselves, especially when nothing is going right in our lives or in the world around us, seems self-evident. However, self-care is not always our first reflex. With the yoni egg practice, you nurture yourself and your energy. You take some time for yourself. Like a thirsty plant being given water, you recover your enthusiasm and joy. This approach requires initial efforts, but regular practice and your desire to do right by yourself will triumph. Over time, new healthy and harmonious habits will become established in your daily life as a woman.

You will give yourself throughout this practice much of the gentleness and love that you most often expect to come from outside sources. Treating yourself with kindness can come one step at a time. Your self-care will grow and one day you will only want to give yourself love. We are not talking about a quest for absolute happiness here but rather a profound desire to treat ourselves well, to grant ourselves attention and time. This will occur naturally over the course of the yoni egg practice. Taking some time for yourself in your active life as a woman will provide many positive results.

Develops Self-Confidence

Self-esteem, self-confidence, and self-assertion are intimately connected. The way you look at yourself, your relationships, and your skills plays a vital role in your self-confidence. It is equally true for your ability to move into action, to leave your comfort zone, and to dare to observe every day so as to learn more about yourself.

> *I have the impression that I gained greater confidence in myself overall. I also experienced heightened feelings during sexual relations, although I have not used the egg all that much up to now.*
> AURÉLIE

> *I regained confidence in myself and in my power to please a man, to no longer just be an object but to be womanly and loved.*
> JEN

The yoni egg, like all regular, positive practices such as meditation, sports, or yoga, makes it possible to become more self-confident. In the interviews I conducted, I heard so many testimonies from different women about the confidence they recovered. Here are a few that might inspire you.

> *I truly feel much more at home in my skin. I have gained confidence about myself and about my life. And I am taking things in hand. I feel like I am a woman without any more expectations. I am in good tone and not alone.*
> BÉNÉDICTE

❝*I feel more confident and more like a woman. I feel a delicious excitement based on improved muscular maintenance.*

GENEVIÈVE ❞

❝*For the time being, I would say that I feel like I am allowed to think of myself as well instead of thinking only about the welfare of others.*

HÉLÈNE ❞

❝*The yoni eggs had a profound effect on me. I think it is difficult to explain in writing. I would have to say that my sense of confidence and relief are the most obvious when I have the egg.*

AXELLE ❞

Reveals the Inner Beauty of Femininity

Having an egg inside you allows you, first and foremost, to establish contact with your yoni, to familiarize yourself with your most intimate domain, and from this to feel "more feminine"—that will allow your inner beauty to radiate.

❝*What is there to say at the end of one month? I have the impression that my egg allows me day by day to accept myself for who I am (it is high time!). I have a new sensation of gentleness and ease when having sex.*

ASTRIDE ❞

Many of us are apt to judge ourselves and compare ourselves with others. We are quick to become jealous and critical of any potential rival. But above all, we are hard on ourselves, as Minke de Vos points out: "Even if a woman is quite beautiful, she will think that her breasts are too small or too big, that her hips are too big or too narrow . . ."

Learning to love yourself is to assert yourself and dare to be unique. The more you learn to love yourself and to accept yourself for who you are, with all your flaws, the more you will glow on the outside.

> 66 I have discovered that we can change things when it is necessary, that we have an absolutely wonderful body that is full of fine surprises, and that the female cycle reveals magnificent treasures that are only asking to be unearthed.
>
> SANDRA 99

Being beautiful goes beyond our appearance. True beauty is established on the inside and radiates to the outside. This is true charisma, the inner power of the woman over herself that magnetizes and seduces so mysteriously. The yoni egg placed inside you, inside your daily life (during a rendezvous, in a meeting, at work, or at lunch), will be carried like a secret—an intimate, centering object whose presence is invisible. You will even forget at times that you are "wearing" it, yet when you need it, your yoni egg will be a powerful ally.

Confidence makes women more feminine and conscious of their inner power and beauty. It may manifest as more sensual for some, while others may feel more able to be vulnerable, open, or seductive. Prompted by the yoni egg, we offer ourselves the love and attention we have come to expect from the outside. In this way, the yoni egg practice allows us to reconnect with and feel the strength that we carry inside of ourselves and that we are now consciously tapping into, allowing ourselves to be confident about our future and talents.

Transforms Your Sexual Energy

As we have seen, yoni eggs work on various aspects of our sexuality, including both the physical and muscular dimension and the energetic and spiritual dimension. As Aisha Sieburth notes:

> The practices as a whole gradually awaken, transform, and refine sexual energy, allowing us to fully experience our intimacy on the

physical, emotional, and spiritual planes. This life energy is precious and sacred, and its healing and creative potential is enormous! We are conceived from sexual cells that contain all the resources of the original DNA to help us achieve our destiny. From a Taoist perspective, sexual energy is the primal matter that is the foundation of the alchemical process that keeps us in good health, transforms our emotions, and encourages spiritual awakening by fully reconnecting to our own source. It takes time to learn and master the techniques and then be in a position to share them with your partner, as much for women as for men.

Even in the early stages of this practice, women witness astonishing changes within themselves and their lives.

> 66 I am in the middle of rediscovering my sexuality with
> the yoni egg. I've been divorced for three years and am
> starting a new chapter of my life. I have met someone.
> My sexuality is clearly more dynamic, more inventive,
> and extraordinary.
>
> JEANNE 99

Reconnecting to your sexual energy and helping it to blossom is one of the big benefits of practice with the egg.

For heterosexual couples, penetration is an important step because it is a threshold. A primordial threshold. It can be an incredible and magical experience. But if we keep on letting in the wrong people, the yoni, which has a highly sensitive energy, will require, over time, very strong penetrations to obtain the slightest sensation or orgasm.

According to Taoist wisdom, as soon as we experience a penetrative sexual act without protection, both partners start entering a very deep karmic level. The heaviest sexual energies that are located in the sex organs carry within them ancestral energies: ancestral chi and all our ancestral karma. This means that all patterns, every-

thing that needs to be healed and transmitted through our lineage, is carried within us as energy.

When we experience full penetration, we have the opportunity to perform a very deep healing. But if we start to open this door to people toward whom we do not feel an enormous amount of love and connection, then all these things that should be healed shall start to blend with our own energy, and new emotions rise to the surface that are not even our own. You will wake up in the morning feeling awkward, and the person you were so intimate with the night before will become a stranger.

Frees Creative Energies

Vital energy, or chi, is the universal life force. This chi can be blocked and stagnant in any part of your body, including your yoni. Wearing your egg will allow you to gently awaken this energy, put it into motion, and make it circulate throughout your entire body. This can create stored emotions to resurface at the early stages of your yoni pratices. Be gentle with yourself, have compassion and nurture yourself in the process. New creative energies will also surface as you let go of your past and expectations. Remember to breathe deeply to oxygenate your entire body and facilate the release of what is no longer yours to carry. A feeling of creativity and freedom will result from such a pratice.

Organically, waves of sexual energy will start to rise more frequently within your body, and the muscles of your yoni will contract gently and freely, allowing more pleasure to flow in and up. The body will express itself more freely, more harmoniously . . . The yoni egg will participate in gradually surrendering to more joy, vitality, and peacefulness.

It is for these reasons that the yoni egg is also called the "energetic egg." Because it gives women access to their innate vitality, the yoni egg provides a lot of energy. The primary practice is to evolve consciously with your yoni egg as you free up stuck emotions and memories. As Jutta Kellenberger says, "When you perform the exercises, you will feel totally energized and galvanized, because it gives us so much life and because there are so many energies stuck inside our yoni." These are energies to which you haven't had access so far. Imagine what you can now create with them.

As Aisha Sieburth explained to me:

The mineral substance of the egg that comes out of Mother Earth is a very noble form of matter that has the power to awaken the "sacred cauldron" of our femininity. This cauldron is a space of creative energies continuously connected to the energy of the Earth— the energy of the trees and all living things that share a connection with our sexual energy—and all are capable of engendering life. We have the power to create life. Isn't that incredible?

This energy, when it is not used to conceive a child, is made available to other life plans—both material and spiritual. The yoni egg gives support to this progression of creation, creativity, and fulfillment by helping us maintain our position as women in the balance of our male and female aspects. Our creative energies are then harmonious.

To some extent the openings are doors through which we can absorb the nourishing energy of the Earth to strengthen our secretory organs and glands. This allows all the flows to circulate to cleanse our inside and then transform and awaken the fire of our sexual energy. This energy, when it has been awakened with the love fire from our heart, connects with the inner space and with the inner smile. And these regions of our glands and organs can receive a nourishment that makes an initial cleansing possible, in connection with the elements of nature.

Liberates Past Memories

The yoni egg will help free much more than your sexual activity, your sense of well-being, and your confidence. All of that in and of itself is already quite a lot, but there is so much more in each of you: your family memories are present in the form of engrams in your yoni. The yoni egg practice can initiate what we will refer to as a "transgenerational" cleansing. According to many teachers, our soul came to Earth at this time to purify itself from limiting beliefs and negative past experiences both in our past lives and in our lineage, so we can shift to a new consciousness on Earth. Aisha explains:

It is inescapable. It is a work of alchemy and transformation. It changes lead into gold—in other words, it transforms all our wounds, all our pains, all the difficulties and obstacles we have been able to construct due to conditioning during our life on Earth. The things left unsaid, beliefs, thoughts, and everything we have inherited from the generations before us that we never talk about. The women who lived before us have bequeathed a sacred burden to us, transmitted from yoni to yoni. That is what is so wonderful.

You should know that here and now, in our own lives, we can undo all these chains of suffering and hardship and help all the women who were here before us thanks to the yoni egg practice. Personally, I did a great deal of in-depth work, a lot of preparation that consisted of getting to know myself and gathering together the maximum quantities of fire and water for my "sacred cauldron."

Respecting your body, honoring the goddess inside and your yoni like a sacred temple, listening to her messages, and recognizing your yoni's wisdom will over time activate new energy centers and activate ancient wisdom you were not conscious of before.

THE POSITIVE EFFECTS ON PERSONAL HEALTH

The primary physical and physiological benefit of the egg, as we have already seen, is a better understanding of our personal anatomy. The insertion of the egg allows you, above all else, to better understand and feel this intimate part of yourself. By acquainting yourself, through the egg, with your yoni and its opening (the large and small lips), you will quickly become aware of any existing tensions.

If you are feeling some small pains or a source of discomfort, explore this part of your body by taking some time to massage your yoni with the stone egg. Vary the pressure, with gentleness, on the outer area of your yoni to release tensions. You might feel emotions emerging on the surface. This comes along with the yoni egg practice when some memories have been stored in our yoni. Take it one step at a time and give yourself conscious love and care. You are not the same woman as you were. You now have the capacity to welcome those emotions, observe them, and thank them for all the teachings they brought in your life. You no longer need to carry them inside your body. Welcome these emotions without judging what has happened. Take advantage of the challenge to be kind to yourself at this moment. While exploring your yoni with the jade egg, do not try to hold back your tears, smiles, or pleasure. Discover the unknown. Let the magic happen. Massaging your yoni with your egg will create a more and more intimate relationship between the two. It takes time, like any relationship. This gentle massage will also have a stimulating and lubricating effect, facilitating the egg's insertion into your yoni. I will talk more about this in chapter 6.

Once inserted, the egg invites new internal sensations. Over the course of time, you will be able to feel the different parts of your vagina as well as its heat and texture. If you keep an open and curious mind, your knowledge of yourself and this part of your body, which so often is still seen as taboo, will lead you to experience a greater sense of fulfillment in your daily life. Little by little, your yoni will no longer hold any secrets for you. It will relax. A relaxed yoni means a more radiant you. You are more conscious, open, and magnetic. Don't take my word for it, test it for yourself.

❝ Use of the egg allowed me to feel the inside of my yoni better, to make myself more aware of it.

FLORENCE ❞

Toning the Perineum

A perineum in good tone is a perineum that is in shape and can be felt!

Equipped with the tone test described earlier (see pages 17–19) and the advice of your doctor or physical therapist, you are now aware that it is important to keep watch of the tone of this area and to take care of it. Being proactive in this regard is best!

> 66 My expectations of the yoni egg involved rehabilitating my vagina, which was very loose even though I never had children, and to see if the egg could help improve a perimenopause that was coming on a bit too early.
>
> ANNE 99

If your perineum is too tight or too loose, if it lacks tone or has too much tension, it will be less sensitive to pleasure, but, more importantly, it will be unable to guarantee the fulfillment of all its functions, which are essential for the body.

Having an ultramuscular yoni is not the goal; in fact, that could even have negative effects such as numbness, pain, and a change in blood flow. So my advice is not to overdo it. Balance your time of practice with time off to observe, and get to know your yoni with and without the egg inside. The more you listen to the messages of your yoni and your body, the more you will know exactly when it is best to use the yoni egg.

> 66 I bought a fairly small egg to rehabilitate my perineum, which had been overly contracted for as long as I can remember.
>
> VALENTINE 99

The objective is first and foremost keeping the perineum well toned so that it prevents any drop of the organs and maintains optimal functioning of the body.

> 66 I saw a very quick improvement in the tone of my perineum, as well as an overall increase in my energy and sense of well-being.
>
> PAULINE 99

The numerous muscles that make up our pelvic floor are to some extent like a hammock that supports our organs. They start at the pubic bone (in the front) and extend to the spinal column (in the back). Just like a hammock, the pelvic floor can become torn or worn out and then sink down, sometimes causing the organs to drop. Urinary incontinence, numbness, vaginal dryness, excessive lubrication, weak libido, pelvic pain, and even a loose vagina can be the consequences of a lack of tone in this portion of our anatomy.

For Aisha Sieburth:

If you wish to begin rehabilitating your perineum, you must first and most importantly have a clear understanding of what the perineum is, where it is located, and how it functions. The perineum is made up of a number of muscles that coexist and work together. These are active muscles. The interaction of this set of muscles allows the proper maintenance of the pelvic floor and its structures. Some tissues (ligaments or fascia) allow the muscles to maintain the organs as well as all the organic structures of the lower abdomen. These muscles as well as the muscles of the perineum control the opening of the vagina, the anus, and the urethra. The pelvic floor muscles as well as those of the lower abdomen are governed and controlled by nerve circuits in the brain and the spinal column. Your health and your physical shape directly depend on the good tone of your pelvic floor! The eggs will help you here magnificently.

The insertion of the egg, which is accompanied by a series of contraction and relaxation exercises, allows the perineum to be toned through the vaginal channel. The use of the yoni egg all through your life as a woman is a core part of finding fulfilled and balanced personal health.

Preventing Organs from Dropping

The pelvic floor depicted on the left on page 31 is weakened and the organs are collapsing and dropping. The depiction on the right allows us to see how firm and toned the vagina is when the pelvic floor is also in good tone.

Keeping our pelvic floor muscles strong and reactive requires regular practice with the yoni egg. But this will not be enough if the drop of the organs is already well advanced. The counsel of a doctor or physical therapist will allow you to know whether you are experiencing organ drop, and then you can act accordingly.

"The drop of organs is often connected to a lack of energy and awareness of the pelvis. All you need to do is awaken the pelvis's energy with pumping motions and lift and bend the sacrum with the perineum, combined with breathing. The yoni egg offers an excellent support for strengthening muscles and ligaments," says Aisha Sieburth.

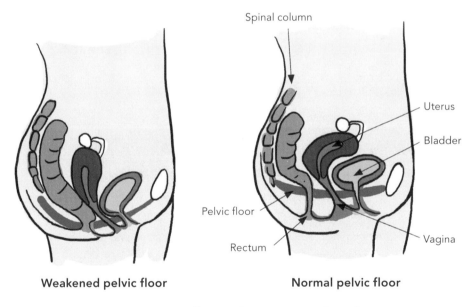

Spinal column

Uterus

Bladder

Pelvic floor

Rectum

Vagina

Weakened pelvic floor   **Normal pelvic floor**

*Figure 3.1. Difference between a weakened
and normal pelvic floor*

Creating Regular Cycles and Providing Relief
from Painful Periods and Premenstrual Syndrome

Premenstrual syndrome (exemplified by groin pain, cramps, stabbing kidney pain, fatigue, breasts feeling like they are ready to explode, headaches, mood swings, water retention, nausea, and diarrhea), painful periods, and irregular cycles are a concern for many women. Thankfully, there are natural solutions, including the practice of the yoni egg, for improving your experience of the cycles.

66 *My basic cycle would last a long time, around forty-five days, and I had heavy periods (I was not taking any form of contraceptive). But since I began using the egg, I have had shorter cycles every month.*

ÉMELINE 99

66 *I now have greater awareness of the muscles of my vagina. My uterus has relaxed. Before it was the core of extremely painful tension (menstrual pains, pains when cuddling, pains when standing or lying down, lumbar pains . . .).*

SOPHIE 99

Aisha Sieburth tells how the yoni egg practice relieved her painful periods.

I had painful periods when I was young. When I discovered this practice with the egg and breast massage, it was a revelation. It was incredible! In the time it took to go from one cycle to the next, I no longer had any discomfort; I no longer experienced any of these symptoms or migraines. My periods became shorter and shorter.

Following is the advice she gives.

The hormonal system will go out of kilter during the cycle when you are facing stress, at the whim of emotions, diet, and the pace of life. . . . These are all factors that can weaken the communication bond between the glands and, little by little, cause the energy in the organs in the pelvis to stagnate and coagulate. As is the case with any blockage, you can get your body moving gently and deeply to release these stagnant energies, get your pelvis back on the right track, and reconnect the glands and their functions by massaging your belly and breasts combined with breathing practices and the yoni egg. These last two practices will get everything back into circulation, tone your sexual energies, and balance your cycles. This will give relief to symptoms due to the stagnation of liver energy caused by overworked glands even at a young age: water retention, breast pains, skin disorders, gastrointestinal problems, nausea, the feeling of something heavy in the pelvic region, headaches, irritability, nervousness, or depression.

The yoni egg should not be used during menstruation. At this time, the yoni needs rest and space to release menstrual blood as optimally as possible, and not stimulation. If you decide to try your yoni egg during menstruation, do not keep it in for any longer than you would a tampon, and take even greater precautions when you clean it so as to minimize risks. I will describe the cleansing of the egg in detail later in the book. But again, it is not recommended by experts to use the egg during this time of the month when you and your yoni need rest.

Preparing to Give Birth

A natural birth is helped by good vaginal muscle tone. When a woman trains with the egg for several months before becoming pregnant, the yoni builds its strength and muscle tone, allowing the woman to master the expulsion of the egg. She will feel more and more mastery, energy, and power for expelling the egg.

Yoni eggs are often pierced so that you can run a string through them and pull on the string, as you would with a tampon, to remove them from the vagina. Many women who have trained with the egg find that they no longer need the string to remove the egg. Their yoni has become more and more flexible, and strong, and they can expel the egg at will. A woman who has trained this way will know how to use her new "yonian" power to facilitate removing the yoni egg at will and giving birth more naturally, possibly as an orgasm.

The use of the yoni egg during pregnancy is a delicate matter. Many experts advise against it. The first three months of pregnancy are risky, and the possibility of a miscarriage is higher. Women who have begun their practice with the yoni egg at least six months before conception and regularly use the egg, are confident about their practice, and feel in tune with their body can, for short intervals, keep using the egg to preserve their connection with their yoni. They can also apply the egg on the tummy and skin for twenty minutes while lying down to connect with and benefit from the stone's properties. They are strongly advised, however, to never wear their egg when sleeping during pregnancy.

THE PREVENTIVE
AND RESTORATIVE BENEFITS

The yoni egg practice can have measurable benefits on the prevention or detection of health problems. There is nothing surprising about this: when you are more attentive to and in tune with your yoni, you will more quickly feel and notice if something is not right, or you will have a better understanding of what the yoni requires to feel better. The egg will help you take better care of your yoni and encourage you to see your doctor or gynecologist whenever you feel it is necessary.

In addition, yoni egg practice can help you to heal more quickly after a serious medical event like a difficult birth or operation. Several concrete examples confirm this.

Hysterectomy
Aisha Sieburth says:

> In the case of hysterectomy (removal of the uterus), you can use the yoni egg (unless they are medically contraindicated). They can even be particularly beneficial as this kind of operation creates a physical and energetic "void" that needs to be filled. The conscious and benevolent practice of the yoni egg can provide a reassuring presence, both physically and energetically, that will support the internal tissues, help them to stabilize, and strengthen hormonal

secretions. This will generate more energy and revitalize and optimize the recovery and healing process.

Rehabilitation after a Difficult Birth

66 *I gave birth and got an episiotomy that became torn and infected—a total catastrophe. No more sensation during sex, a leaky bladder . . . sucks when you are thirty years old! My homeopath advised me to try some "alternative methods." I invested in a yoni egg, which worked wonders for me!*

LAURENCE 99

Detecting the Presence of Fibroids

66 *During the first week, the egg allowed me to sense a point of unexplainable discomfort. I made an appointment with my gynecologist, who discovered an old fibroid the size of a golf ball. I was so thankful that my use of the yoni egg helped me detect it.*

BRIGITTE 99

Urinary Incontinence

According to the U.S. Department of Health and Human Services Office on Women's Health, urinary incontinence affects twice as many women as men and more than 4 in 10 women sixty-five and older. This incontinence can be due to pregnancy, childbirth, menopause, stress, and age. A small amount of urine is released involuntarily during a sneeze or a cough or as a result of a physical or athletic effort. This can affect even very young women after they have given birth. Many more women become easy prey to this disorder because of the weakening of their muscles.

In all cases, urinary incontinence due to physical exertion is the result of the relaxation of the urinary sphincter (the muscle that snugly holds the urethra and closes the bladder) or the loosening of the muscles of the perineum. Exercises with the yoni egg make it possible to strengthen the muscles of the pelvic floor so that the bladder remains securely in place and the urethra fully sealed. If the exercises with the egg are performed on a regular basis, improvements will appear. If the large yoni egg doesn't stay inside of you, there is a good chance you need to get professional help. The yoni egg will help you maintain and possibly increase your yoni powers once you have been medically helped. It is important to take this matter seriously. Like any other muscle, those of the pelvic floor must be worked regularly to remain strong.

SEXUALITY AND LIBIDO

Stimulation of Vaginal Lubrication and Hydration

Because it is still a taboo subject, vaginal dryness is rarely mentioned by women. This condition often leads to an uncomfortable burning sensation or discomfort during the sex act. It is connected to a loss of vaginal hydration and lubrication. These two phenomena are independent but intimately connected for women.

Osteopath Corinne Léger explains that

vaginal hydration is the natural moisture of the vagina. The flow of lubrication is triggered by sexual arousal: it is an additional source of moisture that occurs through the pores of the vaginal mucous membrane.

She adds:

The yoni egg will improve natural hydration as well as encourage lubrication. If vaginal dryness is an issue, it is advised to use a natural cream or coconut oil to promote better external lubrication of this intimate part of the body, which will help with introducing the egg into the vagina. Wearing the egg and performing the exercises will then help achieve better vaginal moisture.

Users have confirmed that the yoni egg has allowed them to improve the lubrication and moistness of their vagina.

> 66 Some time after I had been wearing the egg, I began
> to have far better lubrication. I began having
> vaginal secretions again, something that had not
> happened since my perimenopause. My periods also
> came back after a six-month absence.
>
> CATHY 99

Invigorating and Rebalancing the Libido

Our libido can be defined as our search for pleasure and sexual desire. Each of us has it, and at some point in our lives we all have to deal with lowered libido. Before we go deeper into this subject, let's be clear that there is no such thing as a "normal" libido or a "normal" sexual rhythm. All the same, your libido can be lessened due to a variety of reasons, including stress, worry, fatigue, pain during sexual relations, illness, and medications.

> 66 With the egg, my libido began to wake up again.
> I had the impression of being reborn. I had separated from
> my partner two years earlier when I thought I had lost it.
>
> DELPHINE 99

Your daily routine can also be responsible for loss of libido. If you're suffering from low libido, it is always helpful to consult a sexologist or specialist to determine whether this situation is new or long-term and whether it is generalized or specifically connected to your partner.

Reinventing yourself, loving your body and your partner's, if you have one, is part of the natural stages of flowering that we experience over a lifetime. Endearments, massages, kisses, pleasures, and the power of touch can be self-administered if you are not getting them from a partner. Either way, your yoni egg could become a powerful tool to harmonize your sexuality as you bring more consciousness to this part of your body.

It is certain that our body speaks to us, and it is also certain that we often do not take the time to listen to its messages. Through the yoni egg practice, women will become aware of the importance of devoting time to themselves to take care of their yoni and to listen to what it has to say to them. The yoni egg allows women to reconnect to themselves through gentle, attentive, and healing gestures.

Aisha Sieburth says:

The yoni egg brings more energy into this part of the body, and suddenly we find our sexual energy renewed. If your libido is a little lacking, this will increase the vibrational level of your body, pleasure, and the frequency of orgasms. It offers a balance between stimulation and relaxation. It is healing in its own right for a woman to feel this. This practice allows us to fill an empty space within ourselves with the power of love and touch.

Many women have experienced an improvement in their libido with the use of the jade egg, because it acts simultaneously on the levels of fulfillment and the release of tension. Your yoni will feel as if it is being heard and understood, and it will guide you toward the next steps, whether they consist of seeing a specialist, finding answers within, or performing the yoni egg exercises on a regular basis. The necessity and power of working on yourself then becomes self-evident. The yoni egg is not an end in itself, but it will contribute to your happiness by helping you obtain a better understanding of your body so that you will be more in tune with your desires and will gain greater awareness of this sacred part of your body and of life.

❝ *My libido is clearly much stronger; my yoni is in much better tone. I feel more like a woman, more anchored too.*

Emily ❞

66 *It made me aware (or rather, it reinforced my grasp of the fact) that my well-being also depends on a vital energy that circulates in my body and that an awakened libido forms part of this process.*

LORIANE 99

Respecting and honoring your yoni like a sacred temple gives you more reasons to celebrate life and to restore a communication—one that may have been lost or possibly never even established—with it.

The egg can also help in cases where your libido is too strong. Aisha Sieburth says, "The fire is out or else it is running wild! In both cases, this is a matter that can spoil or improve life, depending on the way you choose to manage it. It is better to learn how to channel your sexual energy rather than being its slave."

Intensifying Orgasms

Foreplay, caresses, positions, breathing, communication, undulation, rhythm, stimulation, and training are all subjects about which orgasms inspire discussion! There are reams and reams of advice available on this subject. How could anyone be against having more orgasms? It is an exceptional moment that releases all the energy of the body, in which the mind stops, in which a person becomes one with life, and in which space and time no longer exist . . . Yes, the orgasm is what most connects us to the universe, to the sensations that some people seek in spirituality, meditation, yoga, or even energy therapies. The seventh heaven is completely accessible and can be made even stronger and more intense, allowing an even greater liberation. So why would we not ask for more?

Tantra expert Shashi Solluna says:

This energy, when it climbs, can open the heart and the mind, and it can rise all the way to the crown. When it does this, we go through this orgasmic experience of dissolving into everything that exists and becoming one with the universe, or rather to remember that we all formed part of the universe. And in my opinion, this is really the great spiritual mystery of sacred spirituality.

There is no magic button for orgasms, nor any technique that works on every body. The way to intensify your orgasms is through having a better understanding of your body, hearing what it is saying, working toward greater relaxation, and striving for the well-known letting go. Nothing is gained from trying to go too fast. "Women are like water. They take time to come to a boil. Men, though, are like fire. They need hardly any time to become stimulated and aroused," Mantak Chia told me at a seminar I organized for him in Paris. Taoist teacher José Toirán added, "And just because we have brought a woman to climax once does not mean that we will succeed the next time by acting the same way!"

But a person does not climax only in bed or during sexual relations. The climax is a way of seeing life and profiting from each moment of life. It is recognizing the best in everything and appreciating, receiving, and taking the time to savor it. This is a true yes to life and to yourself!

❝ *I have an orgasm when I am wearing the egg and caress myself. It is like a tsunami.*

SOPHIE **❞**

❝ *I am trying to gain a more fulfilling sexuality, to be able to "come" in every sense of the word, to be in greater harmony with my body (and my soul, which goes together with it, in my opinion).*

PERINNE **❞**

From the Clitoris to the Brain

The different interviews about sexuality that I have done over the past eight years have taught me that there are several types of orgasm: the clitoral orgasm, the uterine orgasm, and the brain orgasm. According to Jutta Kellenberger, "The majority of women have trouble reaching orgasm. Others manage to have a clitoral orgasm, but they do not feel anything on the inside of their yoni. When it comes to orgasms of the uterus and brain, most women have never experienced them."

She goes on to explain that "when the energy begins circulating, it climbs up toward the heart and then toward the brain like a fountain." Once the clitoral orgasm has been mastered, you must start working on the uterine orgasm, also called "womb orgasm." This is a sacred orgasm because it can be accompanied by the female ejaculation, which is a great emotional liberation, a cleansing, and a release of memories. The yoni egg practice will prepare women for these stages as they progressively explore more secrets the yoni has to reveal.

Sexual Fulfillment at All Ages

The pornographic industry and the billions of dollars it generates have desacralized sex, making it empty and most often denigrating or dehumanizing to women. José Toirán explains to us what caused his personal evolution that led him to quit the pornography industry after seven years and to pursue the profession of sexual healer and coach.

> I had to learn how to hold back my ejaculation. The scenes were never-ending, and I could not ejaculate when I wanted. There was nothing natural about this. Everything was calculated and filmed so that it seemed like the orgasms and scenes were real, but they were not. Many people ended up doing drugs, became neurotic, had serious health concerns, and underwent other atrocities. They were snagged in the trap of money and power. The pornography industry and the billions of dollars it generates continue to do a lot of damage.

To measure up to porn stars is not conceivable, feasible, or desirable, even with stimulants. Jutta Kellenberger reminds us that

> sexuality is connected to our vital energy. It is not something separate or apart. When our vital energy is low, we need coffee and

stimuli because we are exhausted and we have to survive until the weekend. People do a lot of things that are rather harmful. They hurt themselves.

Contrary to some, José evolved in his profession and chose to quit porn thanks to the tantric and Taoist practices that he would end up teaching all over the world.

I learned of the studies of Mantak Chia and his books that taught how to have orgasm without ejaculation. This was a real revelation to me. I had never imagined that the body had this ability. A new life and a deeper learning process allowed me to offer my skills to women and men so that they could learn a new way to experience their sexuality, differently from what they had learned from the pornography industry or painful personal experiences.

He went on to say:

Everything can be fixed. We are not condemned to live with our limiting experiences. I am convinced that healing is possible for everybody. It is not humane to live with such limiting, constraining memories for the rest of your life.

Women are rediscovering their bodies and a more fulfilling sexual experience at all ages of life. It has become a ritual, a moment of blossoming, joy, and freedom. Pleasure, orgasm, libido, and energy are continuously unfolding toward celebrations that, beyond the pleasure they give, offer meaning. This begins with a better understanding of the yoni, of its sensations and of what gives it pleasure, as well as with greater respect for yourself and the sexual act itself, as depicted by Shashi Solluna.

If you have a sacred temple that has been magnificently decorated, you do not want someone to come into it in mud-covered boots.

You expect that the people who enter it will wash themselves before going inside. They will bow and give it reverence before the gates of the temple open.

Over the course of her life and during her practice with the yoni egg, a woman will desire relations with partners who respect her, who will take their time and adapt themselves to the goddess she is, in order to allow the doors of her yoni to express the immense gratitude she will feel for having lovers who honor its fragility, beauty, power, and softness. This will be a new beginning.

> **"** *I allowed myself to be completely flooded by carnal pleasure. My sexuality was improved, but, most importantly, the way I looked at my own body had become gentler. The most surprising thing was my wardrobe . . . I allowed myself to wear clothes that seemed sexier yet respectful of the goddess within.*
>
> JULIE **"**

Initiating Young Women into Their Bodies and Their Sexuality

The importance of living a life of fulfilled sexuality is not often freely shared with younger people. When discovered via images and videos distributed on the internet, a woman's body will not give a man all its capabilities of bliss and pleasure, and she will not find the deep satisfaction she is looking for so intensely.

Learning to know your body, its vital energy and its inner beauty, and to transmit its secrets from woman to woman, from one generation to the next, are traditions and knowledge that have become lost. In some parts of the world, women gather together with other women, and men with other men, accompanied by an instructor, to receive an education in sexuality and to discover its sacred nature. Once upon a time in Asia, both men and women pursued their own forms of practice. Before looking for a partner, a woman spent a great deal of time massaging her own breasts, using the jade egg, and a good many other things to open her own energy body and activate it. Shashi Solluna laments:

Now, during adolescence, teenagers are in a hurry to find someone who will give them something, and they often meet someone who, on the energy level, has absolutely no idea what they are doing. Everyone is clumsily stammering, and, generally speaking, there is not very much energy activation. On the level of intimacy, every-thing has become fairly chaotic, a shambles, a shit show. It is a shame that we have lost the places of education, the temples where people went when they were adolescents to learn how to work with their energies. There are so many different forms of energy that are activated at this age, but nobody really has any clue about how to channel them. When you are basing yourself on this, you really want to wait, you want to be able to connect to the other person on sev-eral different levels. You want to put the personalities together, the energies together, dance together, play together, breathe together, and also spend time together in nonsexual intimacy, to kiss and touch and caress each other, and wait for the body to tell you, "Yes, we can go there now."

The yoni egg will allow even the youngest women to discover their bodies by taking the time to caress and massage themselves with the egg. It will give them the opportunity to lift the veil that conceals the outer and inner secrets of their yoni and thereby discover sexuality in accordance with their own bodies.

THE EGG IS ALSO GENEROUS FOR MEN AND FOR COUPLES!

For Men

Did you know that we women are not the only ones who can benefit from the practice of the yoni egg? Men can also feel the effects of the transformation of our yoni on several levels.

Right away, there is a direct benefit for men. When the tone of a woman's perineum is strong and she can control her vaginal contractions, she is able to make love better with a man. And men truly love to make love with a woman whose yoni is totally toned, as it gives them even more delicious sensations. Making love to a woman with a somewhat loose vagina offers them fewer sensations. The experience will be more ordinary. As Mantak Chia says, "The best way to keep a man is to have your vagina fully toned!"

On this subject, Taoist massage (*chi nei tsang*) expert Shashi Solluna, who was trained by Mantak Chia, told me during an interview that

when you train with the jade egg, after a while your body will begin to contract in the same way it contracts when making love with a man. As a woman, it is as if you were training the walls of your vagina to be able to do this, and this entices a man. All of this part of the body is drawn into the interior. It is very intense, very amazing, and very strong for the man to feel this. And it is also felt this way by the woman, because it uses all the muscles of her vagina, not just some of them. There are an enormous number of sensations, and it provides a great deal of pleasure.

Aisha Sieburth develops this aspect further.

When we are making love with our loved one, that is the time when we can give ourselves that ability to intermingle, to awaken the orgasmic vibrational rate to its maximum extent to have an orgasm not only with our sex organs but also with our glands, our other organs, our entire spinal cord. The result of a sexual relation is not only orgasm but also nirvana and longevity, if practiced according to the Taoist practices taught by Mantak Chia.

For the Couple

Performing exercises with your egg allows you to squeeze your vagina more effectively and therefore have better control and feel more pleasure. The intensification of the orgasms allows a couple to cultivate a delicious intimate life filled with pleasure. Practicing together encourages the fulfillment of both partners to happen more quickly.

Because many women find themselves pursuing their spiritual journey alone, the egg will provide an opportunity to share a tool that can challenge their partner differently and help them open up! A number of you have confided to me that you do not talk about your egg to your spouse. If you want these magical moments to remain yours alone, keep your practice secret, but if it is only because you don't dare, even though your heart is telling you to talk about it, go for it! You may be pleasantly surprised at the welcome your egg will receive. Some delectable moments can result, as I will explain when describing the ritual for couples in the final chapter of this book. Watching you practice ritualizing your yoni eggs in front of his eyes could change your partner's perception of what makes you happy. A new adventure could begin. Whether you are in a relationship with a man or a woman, your partner will appreciate the change and discover your new intimate explorations! Exciting for most!

" *My partner reacted really well. He encourages me to discover my femininity. He has even managed to guess when I'm wearing it (he can tell by my mood).*

ÉMELINE "

" *I felt its benefits with a partner who had also been awakened to the practice of mindful sexuality.*

BEA "

Have confidence and speak to your partner without feeling embarrassed. You might be surprised by his or her reactions and how tuned in to it he or she is. This is something many women have told me, including one who told me that her man was very mechanical in making love to her. One day she showed him how she was using her yoni egg. She took her time with gentleness and love toward her body. Since then her man has been making love to her in a way that is providing her with so much more pleasure by gently listening to her yoni's needs!

It may take a while for the man's interest in the yoni egg practice to appear. For two of the women I interviewed, Nath and Sophie, the egg ended up causing their relationships to evolve with regard to the changes that occurred in their femininity.

> " I did not talk about it with my spouse; he is a huge skeptic. But I noted that his pleasure had increased (we have been in love for twenty-five years). He has still not asked any questions!
>
> NATH "

> " My partner (we have been together for thirty years, and he is the father of my two daughters) eventually became delighted with my enthusiasm. He was truly happy for me . . . and for himself (!) . . . even if the whole thing was a little (or even completely!) inexplicable to him.
>
> SOPHIE "

PART TWO

How to Choose the Perfect Yoni Egg for You

4

The Egg Adapts to All Stages of a Woman's Life

The yoni egg is adaptable to all ages and all lifestyles, from the most sexually active women to those who have lost all desire for sex. It can be employed by women to help them discover their body, recover their self-confidence, and restore tone to their perineum, and it can offer a seductive magnetism. The reasons we use the egg will differ depending on our particular circumstances, needs, and intentions, and the size and type of stone used will differ for each of us.

AT THE PEAK OF YOUR SEX LIFE

At that time in our lives when we feel most confident, when we begin to know who we are and therefore to fine-tune what we want and sublimate our desires, when we are able to make good choices about our partners and know what our yoni wants or doesn't want—that is the ideal moment for engaging in the egg practice. Even at this stage of our lives, there is still a lot we need to discover about ourselves. The yoni egg offers a golden opportunity for continuing to liberate our creative energy, find our power, assert our sexual energy, and follow the teachings of our yoni.

We pursue this energy to co-create our lives in a positive and proactive way. Your pleasure will increase with greater mastery of your body and your orgasms, and you will be able to gain access to dimensions of yourself that were unknown or only barely glimpsed before. The time will have come to express the sacred feminine hidden inside you. You can then abandon yourself completely to your intuition to choose the egg that will be best suited to your needs, and with it you will be in a position to prepare for the next steps in your journey of self-discovery.

"Playing the Flute"

Over time, some women will discover the pleasure of "playing the flute" with their yoni. Yes, you heard me right! But it is not quite the flute or the tune you are probably thinking of! I am referring here to experiments that you and your partner can do that create amazing orgasms by using the muscles of your yoni, without moving, to create simple, light pulsations.

This advanced technique, which might appear complicated in the beginning, is taught by Mantak Chia. It consists of moving your awareness and the egg into the three parts of the vagina: the set of muscles at the opening of the yoni, a middle zone where your egg will often naturally place itself, and the zone at the top near the cervix. It goes without saying that learning this practice requires a great deal of patience, but it is very effective. You start with a large egg and work your way down to a small one.

For my naughtier readers and those who have more sexual demands placed upon them, the egg will allow you to regain your balance and revive your partner if he becomes overwhelmed by your energy. You are entirely free to choose how and for what purposes you will use your egg. It can allow you to feel better control over your yoni, to vary the forms of foreplay, or even to manage certain unsatisfied desires.

For example, Carine uses the egg to help her channel her sexual energy.

66 *When my libido is high, it is quite helpful.*

CARINE 99

Dorothée's practice with the egg has evolved as her goals have changed.

66 *My first objective was to strengthen my perineum,*
but now I use it as a sex toy.

DOROTHÉE 99

FOR WOMEN WHO ARE SINGLE

Being single is not always easy to manage; society does not always view single women kindly, and being single can cause you to doubt yourself and your own power. And if you are single and looking for love, the yoni egg will be of great support. I recommend wearing it for dates! It will give you a sense of mystery and self-love so that you are not looking to get those things filled by your date. It will make you present, aware, gentle, and naturally who you are, without overdoing it (as we can all do when we are nervous or not confident). You will shine from the inside out, and that is sexy! And if you are not looking for a partner, the yoni egg will bring you a gentle presence and support in your daily life. You will feel even more self-content!

Whatever your perspective on being single, live this time of your life to the fullest, do what gives you pleasure, fall back in love with yourself, and be good to yourself! Take advantage of this time to redis-cover and reconnect with yourself. This will make you even more ready to open yourself to new encounters, find fulfillment, and feel your own personal magnetism. Thanks to the egg, you will be fully enmeshed in your femininity and receptiveness, without feeling any need to fall into the arms of the first person to come along and express his or her desire for you. I have personally noted that I no longer attract the same kind of men I did before I started the yoni egg practice and that I am making great strides toward the love of my life. When I wore my yoni egg during the day and during dates, I had the sensation that my energy was being "recycled inside me"; it was no longer leaking away and being shared with everyone around me. By centering myself this way, I gained confidence, autonomy, and sensuality. I became more attractive to and attracted gentle men who where genuinely interested in me for who I was and not for sex only.

And I was not the only woman to experience this phenomenon with the yoni egg during a period of celibacy.

> " I gained greater awareness of my body, and I felt more like a woman. From now on it will be easier for me to have a partner; I just know it. It had been difficult for me to keep a relationship; something was destroyed and I did not know what it was. With the egg I feel much more comfortable in my body.
>
> CATHERINE "

> " I am single. After two months of practice, I no longer used the egg in the same way. I am more in tune with my body and with its incredible energetic sensations. It is more than sexual, and yet I know my body quite well, being an adept of masturbation.
>
> MARIE "

> " I am single, and with the egg I now feel much more 'alive' and much more connected to my sacred feminine. I am in better tone and more conscious about this part of my body. I had a hysterectomy after I had cancer, and because of that, there is a suture at the tip of my vagina.
>
> CÉLINE "

FOR SEXUAL FULFILLMENT

For many women the egg represents a way to reconnect with their bodies and release certain stored memories and energies that have a tendency to extinguish their ardor and desire. It also allows them to rediscover (with the rituals described in later chapters) the beauty and stimulation of the body. Sexual fulfillment will return with practice, accompanied by new ideas and movements that will contribute, if it is what you are looking for, to a sexual rebirth.

Jutta Kellenberger explains:

A woman who has not had any sexual relations for a long time will probably have a lot of tension inside her vagina; she might not have had enough opportunites to get energy circulated in this part of her body. In this case, the skin can become extremely sensitive, so when you begin doing the exercises with the yoni egg, you might feel some minor irritation of the skin or some small pains here and there, and this will call for courage. This is a real commitment, a desire to be seized. You must overcome all these things to open new doors.

" It is undeniable that my sexuality has improved thanks to using the yoni egg. . . . My vagina is in much better tone and more often desire is not found wanting.

SOPHIE **"**

If you want to put the color back into your desires and your sexuality, take the time to choose the size of the egg that suits you best. Trust in your own judgment, or try the different sizes—you will see which works best for you!

" I first bought a large egg because I had not had any sexual relations for a long time. I regretted it because it was too big, and I only used it once. I should have trusted my intuition, which told me to buy the smaller size.

ANNE-CLAIRE **"**

THE YONI EGG FOR
A BUSY, STRESSFUL LIFE

Stress is one of the great scourges of modern life. We are always in a hurry. Between our jobs, families, and the needs of daily life, we never stop running. If a few problems get added to our already jam-packed schedule, it's a disaster.

If you are working, if you have children, if you are not getting enough sleep, if you have a household to run and a relationship to cultivate, stress can quickly soar, as we all know. Taking time for yourself, practicing the yoni egg exercises, taking a walk in nature, meditating, breathing, and working on yourself will guide you along the path of inner calm and relief. With the yoni egg practices, every woman can rediscover her center of balance and determine how the rituals, as I explain them in this book, best work for her to restore meaning to a stressful life.

❝ *With the yoni egg, I have more trust in my status as an independent, entrepreneurial woman as well as a woman who is artistic, sensual, sexual, and vulnerable. My libido has also improved.*
AMÉLIE ❞

Wearing the yoni egg gives us a moment of tenderness, which is lacking in the lives of many women, as can be seen in the case of Lucie.

❝ *The comfort of the jade egg, by its shape, color, and texture, responds precisely to the change I am making in myself, one that tends toward more gentleness and kindness toward myself.*
LUCIE ❞

During an interview I had with Jutta Kellenberger, she touched on an important point connected to all the disorder of our time and all the benefits the egg can provide to help us get free of it.

Exercise with the yoni egg forms a part of some major female practices that allow us to bring the mind's attention into the ovaries, and this is something we need when we are suffering from infertility or having trouble conceiving—in other words, when the womb, in traditional Chinese medical terms, is too "cold." It is then necessary to bring chi into the womb and into the uterus to restore warmth. The egg exercise encourages the focalization of energy toward the lower regions. The problem in our Western societies is that we are no longer slaves (that's a good thing!): we are educated, we go to universities, and we learn lots of things, and therefore all the energy is directed upward, toward the head, and not enough goes toward the bottom. This is why many Western women can no longer conceive and men have less and less sperm: it is because we are too much in our heads! It makes us crazy. We are no longer there [she points to her yoni]. We are no longer in our body, but to conceive a child, we should *be there; the energy should be there, in the lower half of the body.*

YONI EGGS AND ATHLETICS

The more athletic among us have told me that they use the smallest yoni eggs, which are customarily used by the experts in the egg practice, to release vaginal tensions. Here again, it all depends on how toned you are and what you know about your body and your yoni!

The most courageous could even try wearing their egg during sports activities. You must pay attention, though; certain movements can make the egg fall out!

> ❝ I shoot with a bow, and when I loose my arrow, this abrupt movement can cause the egg to fall out. Women need to be warned about certain athletic movements. I might sometime test it on horseback, but I have not yet dared to do so.
>
> Léa ❞

The egg fits in fairly well with sports practices, whether dynamic or gentler, as long as the woman takes some simple precautions. However, avoid using it when biking, running, or horseback riding. For yoga, meditation, and Pilates, the yoni egg will add a nice touch to your practice. Remember to always listen to your body's sensations, so if it hurts or it bother you, remove it.

> ❝ I use it frequently when doing my Pilates.
> CATHY ❞

> ❝ I often do my meditation while wearing my egg.
> EVA ❞

Sexologist and psychotherapist Lara Castro advises athletes who started high-level sports activities at a young age, "You need to work even harder on your perineum. Many great sportspeople, even when very young, have had problems with incontinence. The solution is not to wear a sanitary napkin. It is crucial to begin quickly restoring the tone of your perineum. The yoni egg is perfect for regularly exercising this part of the body."

TRANSITIONAL PHASES AND TIMES OF REFLECTION

During times of change in your life, it is easy to lose confidence in yourself and question the choices you have made. No results are yet visible, you are not always sure which way to turn, and you feel as if you have lost your operating instructions. Everything needs to be rebuilt, and you can find yourself, at times, alone and destitute. Returning to your self and to your body is a first step for regaining contact with your inner wisdom and find the impetus you need to cross through your doubts and fears and make new decisions from a place of joy.

66 *Every day, once I had put the egg in place, I had a better connection with my vagina, which I learned to love! I changed my life, and perhaps the egg helped me. I changed my profession; I now teach yoga, and the egg fits perfectly into this dynamic.*

AURORE 99

The yoni egg practice and its rituals can help you return to yourself, to look back over your life, to observe yourself and understand the road that you have taken up to this point. They can allow you to to get centered again within yourself, to give yourself the time you need and make it available to your body as well, and to take advantage of this moment. They will let you, like Roxanne, discover a new phase of life.

66 *Currently, I am taking stock of the fifty years I've been alive. I am realizing that I have not lived my life the way I wanted. I therefore have a desire to take my life back into my own hands. I should learn how to know myself better, and the egg permits me to concentrate solely on myself as well as on my sacred feminine.*

ROXANNE 99

YONI EGGS, VIRGINITY, AND YOUTH

Countless mothers have asked me how old a young girl should be before starting the yoni egg practice. One thing is sure; introduction of the egg should be undertaken in accordance with the physiological development, maturity, and questions that a young girl has about femininity and sexuality.

Before answering this question, let's take a rapid anatomy lesson on virginity. The hymen is a more or less flexible, delicate, and resistant membrane located at the entrance of the vagina, about one-third to one-half inch behind the labia minora. It has a small opening that allows the blood from menstruation to pass through, and a young girl can therefore use a small tampon or stick her finger inside while leaving this membrane intact.

Rupture of the hymen is commonly associated with the loss of virginity. However, the hymen can also be stretched or broken during childhood as a result of playing sports or other vigorous activity or due to some kind of impact, without the young girl realizing that this has occurred. There are even some women who are born without a hymen, and others whose hymen will not be broken during their first sexual relations. Here again, we note that every woman has a very different yoni; hence the importance of learning as much as possible about this particular part of *your* body and honoring it when you are young.

So, losing your virginity is not solely defined as the loss of this membrane during your first sexual experience. Instead, making love with a partner for the first time is an important initiatory passage in the life of a woman. The respect and love associated with this passage will be even stronger if the young woman is aware of what her yoni wants and doesn't want.

As far as the yoni egg practice is concerned, if a young woman is fully developed (if she has had her first period) and if she has been wearing tampons or menstrual cups during her periods, it will be possible for her to use a yoni egg. The main thing is to make a wise choice regarding the size and material of the egg.

If the young woman feels like she is ready to make first contact with this intimate region and explore it, the egg will be her best friend. A small egg made from rose quartz is ideal for beginners because this magnificent mineral offers a gentle, calming, reassuring energy. It provides a feeling of security and encourages trust. It helps develop self-esteem.

Taking your time and taking things in stages is what Saida Desilets, an expert in the yoni egg practice in the United States, recommends.

First try to perform the exercises using only your imagination (an imaginary yoni egg), and then while using your finger, before moving on to the yoni egg. In the beginning, the most important thing is to understand the way you treat your body, so it is preferable to begin with a feeling of deep respect and curiosity and to pursue it like an experiment without aiming at any specific goal. By going slowly and establishing a relationship with your body, you will form positive neuronal pathways that are filled with pleasure. They will improve your sensual and sexual experiences for the years to come. Let me repeat: take it slowly! Why rush it?

She goes on to note that "for young women whose hymen has not been broken and who want to keep their virginity for their first sexual relationship, the egg practice may well be contraindicated."

But even in this case, a person can start by an initial external approach, as Saida Desilets notes.

It is then preferable, in the very beginning, to save the egg for outside use on the perineum and the vulva, without putting it in. As an initiation in using the egg, it is a good start for becoming aware and discovering this part of the body.

CONTRACEPTIVE METHODS THAT ARE RESPECTFUL OF THE BODY

We saw in chapter 3 how the practice with the yoni egg helps in preventing painful periods and with approaching childbirth more calmly, as well as other moments in the life of a woman and her personal health. The more subtle and expanded awareness of our body that the yoni egg engenders is also an advantage when it comes to selecting appropriate birth control. It is important, of course, to consult a qualified health care professional, but a woman who practices with the yoni egg will have a greater sense of autonomy in relying on her own inner wisdom; she will have a more intuitive grasp of what is good for her body and for her yoni.

The yoni egg can be used in conjunction with any form of birth control, whether the pill, spermicide, implants, injectable contraceptives, male or female sterilization, a male or female condom, IUD (intrauterine device), diaphragm, contraceptive patch, periodic abstinence, or even the vaginal ring. Osteopath Corinne Léger, who herself uses the egg, explains:

There are no contraindications for a woman using contraception in terms of also using a yoni egg. It may even give her the desire to tune in more naturally with her body and to be open to a different contraceptive method, one that is closer to nature and therefore more respectful of her body.

There are precautions to take with some forms of contraception during the use of the egg. With an IUD, for example, it is not recommended to use an egg that has a hole drilled horizontally through it (most eggs are pierced vertically, as we will discuss later).

The vaginal ring, meanwhile, should be taken out during the time you are wearing the egg. Lara Castro says:

The ring can be removed from the vagina for at least three hours and still retain its contraceptive effectiveness. After you finish the yoni egg practice, rinse the ring in cold water and replace it in the vagina within this time frame.

PREPARATION FOR GIVING BIRTH

If you are pursuing practice with the yoni egg, preparation for childbirth need not be limited to toning and softening the perineum and vagina, even though this is a very important contribution. Regular practice can even help make giving birth a true moment of pleasure.

The image that we have of childbirth is still too strongly connected to suffering, pain, and moans. As the author of *La Maternité au féminin* [Maternity from the woman's perspective], Isabelle Chalut says:

The birth of my children was an important turning point in my life. I experienced the medical domination of women in childbirth, and it revolted me. This incredible event that is the birth of a living being has become a painful and potentially dangerous experience. Women find themselves reduced to their uterus, which must be kept in check. Women who speak of experiencing childbirth according to their vision, in tune with their body and their needs, who want to move and yell, who refuse to take an epidural, often still find themselves treated as "misfits." I have attended a fair number of births, and I have seen women completely disconnected from their bodies. The sole possible way out for them when suffering so intensely was the epidural, so they would not feel anything. There is no respect in our society for children's knowledge of what their bodies need. When they reach adulthood, they inevitably find themselves cut off from a part of themselves.

This nurse, who practiced her profession for more than twenty-five years in France, Switzerland, and Quebec and has become a specialist in obstetrics over the past ten years, invites us to listen to our bodies and rediscover our inner wisdom.

If you have a pain in your belly, are you able to tell precisely which organ is affected? What is the cause of this pain? Perhaps you have lost the intimate connection that can tell you what is taking place inside of you at every minute. There are a variety of corporeal approaches that will allow you to recover this subtle hearing that is the basis of this process for becoming autonomous. It is important to know yourself, to relearn how to listen to yourself and to respect what you are feeling inside.

Corinne Léger encourages the use of the egg in this sense:

A natural birth is when, as the birth process begins, the uterus under the effect of the hormones pushes the baby toward the outside, head first. When a woman has worked with the egg for several months or several years before becoming pregnant, the vagina will have become flexible, supple, and in good tone. This is why women who give birth naturally experience it as an orgasmic experience.

YOUNG MOTHERS

The baby has arrived and a new life has begun. Should you be helping your body and yoni to regain a new harmonic consistency after the ordeal of childbirth? Of course, as we have seen, the egg will find its place perfectly in the process of rehabilitating the perineum. Even better, it will help you psychologically and energetically to become the new woman you wish to be.

Following is some extremely valuable advice from Corinne Léger.

The egg practice helps revitalize women who have just given birth and are receiving postpartum care. I would advise starting with a large egg, and as the perineum regains strength, you can move down to a midsize stone. Wait six weeks before starting your practice. It is crucial following the birth that you are certain the tissues are healed in the event of an episiotomy or tearing of the perineum before even imagining starting your practice with the yoni egg again. You should wait for the gynecologist to give you the green light after having checked the condition of your cervix. Once this hurdle has been passed, the yoni egg can be an essential asset for the recovery of your perineum, in combination with the standard rehabilitation procedures. Every woman will find her own practice rhythm and the time she needs to give herself these intimate rendezvous with herself.

The testimonies of Marion and Elizabeth, two young mothers who sent me their testimonials, perfectly describe the various facets of the egg's benefits following childbirth.

❝ *After the birth of my daughter, I went into a huge depression. I felt utterly lost, with a complete absence of any sensations during sex. After three months using my yoni egg on and off, I began feeling sensations—it was super motivating! But more importantly, the vision I had of myself had also changed. It is necessary to regain confidence [after childbirth], and I think that the egg is more effective than physical therapy for this!* ❞
MARION

❝ *When I began getting results, my physiotherapist advised me to do fewer sessions with him and to continue using my yoni egg to 'hold on' to the progress I had made. Today, I wear it three times a week, at minimum. I make a game out of making it move around.*

ELIZABETH ❞

PERIMENOPAUSE AND MENOPAUSE

Perimenopause and menopause are often accompanied by vaginal dryness and a loss of libido. The vagina wall becomes very thin and dries out. But this is not an irremediable situation. I can't tell you that using the egg will bring your yoni back to the condition it was in when you were twenty, but definite improvements can be expected in terms of comfort during sexual relations and with regard to tone.

This is quite clear to Corinne Léger, as she notes:

It is highly recommended for menopausal women to employ the exercises with the egg; it will help them develop greater awareness of a gynecological nature that is often shoved to the side. At this stage of life, the egg practice needs to be connected to a person's innermost self. The individual needs to develop a more subtle way of listening to her body and becoming sensitive to her sacred femininity. It will stimulate the first chakra. At this stage, some women will encounter a problem with vaginal dryness or a loss of tone in the perineum, or both. A regular practice, every day, will allow you to tone and stimulate the pelvic hammock, which can become stretched out due to pregnancies, because of age, or simply because of neglect of this zone that is so extremely important as the foundation of our spinal column. For some women, this will be just what they need to energize their libido!

Menopause is not always what we are told it is, as the yoni egg practice shows for those who use it regularly. The jade egg can help us break free from false ideas and depictions of this stage of life. Aisha Sieburth shows no hesitation when attacking these clichés about menopause.

Menopausal women believe what their doctors are telling them: "You are no longer ovulating, so your sex life is completely shot." I personally really like the image of an anemone, which, through its roots, has pumped out and will suck in and gradually put into circulation the vital force it holds inside. It is this reconnection made possible by the yoni egg that allows menopausal women to get their libido up and running again.

She explains:

The Taoists call menopause the "second spring." It is a sacred moment when the energies that have been deployed through menstruation are now going to be conserved and recycled into the body's tissues to feed the woman's sacred fire. To live this transition fully, all your feminine "flowers" should bloom with greater stimulation of the hormone glands with the jade egg practice, accompanied as always by massaging your breasts, which will awaken the bond between all the glands. The symptoms, such as hot flashes, dizziness, dryness, loss of libido, and insomnia, can be due to the leakage of energy and the drying out of fluids in the upper and lower regions of the body.

Béatrice, from whom I received a testimonial when she was fifty-six and going through menopause, seemed totally content with her yoni egg practice, which helped her be the woman she wanted to be at this stage of her life.

" *After long years with no sexual activity and at the
threshold of life as part of a couple again, I was guided
toward the yoni egg. I was able to reopen the door of my sacred
feminine. . . . I was scared that I would be unable to
physically welcome this man for whom I had been waiting so long.
It took me three days before I was able to insert the small egg,
and then five days for the midsize one.*

BÉATRICE "

FOR MORE DELICATE SITUATIONS

The yoni egg has restorative powers. It takes its place inside of us discreetly and quietly, and then it goes to work. Not by itself, of course. It works as part of a team consisting of you, your yoni, and your egg. In this way it brings together many resources to address the repair of or resistance to trauma. Whether that trauma falls into the context of serious gynecological issues, a birth that proceeded poorly, or a sexual trauma, our yoni and our fundamental energy will find a precious ally in the egg for rebuilding ourselves and moving beyond what we were to become better individuals.

Following a Miscarriage, Stillbirth, or Infant Death

Isabelle sent me the following poignant testimony.

" *The egg is a 'sacred' object for me. Twenty years ago
I carried a baby in my belly for nine wonderful months of love;
unfortunately, this little baby did not want to live in our
earthly world. I have had two wonderful children since then.
Next a fibroid developed inside me that was so
large that the doctor was obliged to remove my uterus.
I chose to use the yoni egg because it filled a void in me.*

ISABELLE "

Isabelle's account is inspiring and so stamped by the truth that it speaks for itself. A miscarriage, stillbirth, or infant death is one of the most painful events in life, both psychologically and physically. Like all traumas, it leaves a mark in your mind as well as in your yoni. You were waiting for your baby with so much happiness, and an accident took her away from you. It takes time and kindness to come back from something like this. The yoni egg will help you cross through this stage and help release these painful memories.

Always listen to your intuition and let your feelings tell you which stone is most suitable for you. After a miscarriage, stillbirth, or infant death, perhaps an egg designed for external use would be more appropriate initially. You must always listen to your body and your yoni to hear what the egg is saying!

After a Hysterectomy

A yoni egg can be helpful after a hysterectomy (unless it has been medically contraindicated). The yoni does not like the physical and energetic void that results from this operation; the egg seeks to fill this void. Aisha Sieburth tells us:

> The conscious and kind practice of the yoni eggs supplies a comforting physical and energetic presence that supports the internal tissues and helps the neighboring organs (especially the intestine) to stabilize. It can take the place of the void left by the missing uterus and truthfully even take up some of the duties the uterus once performed. It will generate more energy to revitalize and optimize recovery and healing.

After Sexual Trauma

Trauma affects us at different levels and, depending on the individual and the stage of life at which it occurs, in different ways. Jutta Kellenberger explains, "When, as a child, someone touches us in a disrespectful manner, or has touched our chest, our immediate reaction is to close ourselves off. A person can close up without it being a major trauma."

In a similar fashion, if, for example, at a very young age a little girl has been given a bath by a man or a woman and felt that man or woman's desire without understanding it, then she will close up and store the memories in her body and in her energy, thereby limiting her potential. Jutta adds, "This blocks the chi as well as blocking the physical plane. The muscles contract. Everybody has their own stories that explain why things are as they are."

After having gone through a traumatic sexual experience in 1994, Saida Desilets now helps women who, like her, have been confronted by life's challenges.

It is a rare woman who has never experienced any sexual trauma. Talking about her traumas is not enough. There is a cellular memory that needs to be released. Some will turn directly to the professionals, but the jade egg will allow most women to do this work by themselves. The reason the egg is so powerful is that, first and foremost, it invites the woman to reconnect with her body and to feel entirely safe while doing so. Next, it allows the cells to be reprogrammed. After having healed my own body from sexual traumas and helped thousands of other women to do the same, I know it is possible to free yourself from the terror and pain of past experiences and to reconnect to your body, to take back ownership of your body, and make it so that pleasure becomes natural again.

Having been the victim of sexual abuse is a very delicate and painful subject for women to deal with, and one that is unfortunately all too frequent.

❝ *I am sixty-two years old, so I took the largest rose quartz egg. I had been subjected to conjugal violence for more than thirty-four years, and I had a hysterectomy when I was forty-two. I want to rediscover my femininity thanks to the egg.*

MARIANNE ❞

❝ *I bought my egg because I suffered from sexual abuse by my father during my childhood. This caused a serious hormonal disease that made me sterile for many years at the very beginning of my life as a woman. It took me six months to work up the courage to put the egg into my yoni. I was apprehensive about it, and I think I needed this whole time of 'ripening' and introspection about myself, and this extremely intimate woman's path in order to do it.*

I then instantly felt complete. I truly had the impression that I was rooted in myself; I felt a lot of inner strength and had finally found my place as a woman on this Earth. It also freed a lot of memories buried in my vagina, my uterus, and my ovaries. With sustained personal work on myself, I was really able, for the first time in my life, to feel free in my femininity, to feel my entire belly and yoni, to be simply freed from the past and freed from these wounds.

I cannot recommend these eggs too highly for all women who have experienced traumas that have attacked their sexuality and integrity. It is an approach for which you have to be ready internally, but I am sure that the egg will arrive when we are ready.

To have this power to liberate female energy that has been trampled down for so long is truly extraordinary, and so important for our time, which is asking women to take back their creative place upon the Earth. You should not hesitate to seek help from a therapist for the release of all these old memories coming to the surface.

ANNE-LAURE ❞

❝ *My egg has calmed the images I carried deep down of violent and degrading sexual relations that had no tenderness or affection. These images had been constantly present for me since the time my sexuality first awoke and never left me until recently; I think this happened thanks to the yoni egg.*

BENÉDICTE ❞

" Until recently (I am almost forty years old) I rarely had happy sex. I was a victim of nonconsensual sex and rapes. I developed a resistance to pleasure. Today, the huge construction site of my life is renewing my connection with pleasure and sharing it with my new companion. This remains a complicated subject for me, and the egg is part of a progression of discovery of myself.

VALERIE "

Forgiving yourself, giving yourself permission to explore sexuality in a different way, regaining your confidence, and finding yourself again demands time with your yoni in order to give it attention and love. It will give you greater guidance and start communicating more and more clearly with you.

The egg, regular practice, your commitment, and your powerful female energy, which may have gone unused until now, will put you on the road to healing. The various experts I met have an abundance of knowledge on all these aspects. Éliane, who is a therapist who also uses the egg, says, "When I meet women who have experienced traumas due to their sex and femininity, I describe the egg to them as a method for really taking a step forward in their inner liberation."

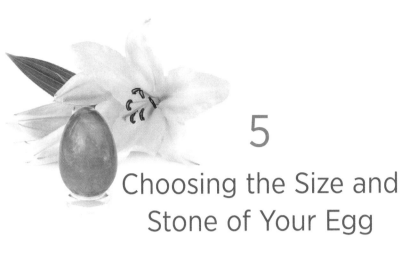

5

Choosing the Size and Stone of Your Egg

Let's talk size—and yes, size does matter! When it comes to yoni eggs, there are three sizes, differentiated by length and width.

Small (which is around 1.6 inches long and 1 inch wide)
Medium (which is around 1.8 inches long and 1.2 inches wide)
Large (which is almost 2 inches long and about 1.4 inches wide)

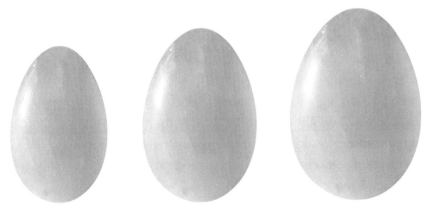

Figure 5.1. Small, medium, and large yoni eggs (actual size)

Like you, your yoni is unique. Remember that it has incredible elasticity, as can be seen when a woman gives birth. Even the largest yoni egg is not as big as an ostrich egg, so there is no call for panic! The large size can seem scary, but it is suitable for a beginning practice for many women. Basically, if the egg is too small, it will not stay in place. It is therefore essential to choose the appropriate size.

The Criteria for Selecting Your Egg

Tone

Advancement in the practice

Age

Athletic activity

Traumas

Surgical operations

Virginity

For most women, the medium and large eggs are ideal.

A young, active woman who has not given birth to children will tend to choose a medium egg.

A woman who has had children by natural childbirth will often have less tone and choose a large egg. Women who are going through menopause or who want to prevent incontinence will also tend to choose a large egg. Keep in mind that if your pelvic floor is flabby, the egg will probably have trouble staying put in your vagina, and your practice should be adapted accordingly (by starting with the exercises of contraction and relaxation while lying stretched out, for example).

After childbirth, many women wait until after their recuperation period to practice the yoni egg exercises. The egg can then help them maintain and improve their progress and also, as I have explained, benefit them on more subtle planes.

Aisha Sieburth advises beginners to choose a large egg.

The important thing, in the beginning, is to have a sensation like this: "Ah! Yes, there, I feel it, I feel a presence that I can really work with." Gradually, through the practice, a person can use an egg that is increasingly smaller and keep it inside without it falling out, even when there is a weight hanging from the string! But it is true that in the beginning it is better to start with something larger.

I would like to point out that, even with a large egg, it is not uncommon not to be able to feel the egg inside you. The golden rule is that if your egg stays inside you, then you have picked the right size. Hence the importance of testing your tone, placing your confidence in your intuition, and carefully reading the contents of this book.

The small egg, for example, cannot stay inside you if you do not have the necessary tone in your perineum. To determine your tone, take the test provided in chapter 2 (pages 17–19). The small egg is also lighter, so it can work in a more subtle way to release tensions in the yoni.

This is why a small yoni egg is recommended for women who have mastered the practice of the yoni egg and the tone of their yoni. But it is also recommended for women who are intensely involved in sports or women whose vaginas are very tight and compressed, so much so that they cannot insert tampons, for example; this situation is sometimes connected to a sexual trauma. The small egg is also recommended for young women who are just being initiated into sexuality and their own bodies.

The small eggs can also be used, with experience, in pairs, as José Toirán suggested during a workshop I arranged for him in Bordeaux. It involves using your vaginal muscles to cause one to go up while the other goes down so as to obtain better mastery of the vaginal rings and therefore of the orgasm.

EVOLVING WITH
THE DIFFERENT SIZES

In addition to these practical recommendations, when you are choosing your egg you should let yourself be guided by your feminine intuition, your desires, and what attracts you most. In fact, size is not the only criterion to take into account when making your selection. Our feminine nature holds its own mystery, and the body knows which egg is intended for it . . . Listen to the little voice of your intuition, or ask your yoni directly. The first response that you feel is often the right one.

Many women choose to acquire three eggs so they can develop their practice. As a general rule, the more you progress in this practice, the better your ability to choose the egg that is calling you. Solla Pizzuto, an expert masseuse, explains this quite simply as follows:

It depends on the woman's anatomy, her structural anatomy, on whether she has had children. There are three sizes: small, medium, and large. In my practice I use all three, and they are all wonderful.

CHOOSING THE STONE

Scientific studies provide us with information on the formation of minerals, their chemical and physical properties, and their composition, but they do not give us a complete picture, lacking vision about the energetic properties of the stones.

Gérard Cazals, author of *La quintessence des pierres* [The quintessence of stones], explains, "The intrinsic energy of the stone, our specific energy needs, and our reactions to the stone's energy will be inseparable factors for clearly grasping the effect that a stone could have on us."

Gemstones and crystals played an important role in ancient civilizations. Today, they are regaining a place in our everyday lives thanks to lithotherapy, which uses gemstones and crystals to help us gradually recover physical, emotional, mental, or spiritual balance. The subtle influence of minerals plays a role in the context of a holistic healing approach, as it touches on all levels of the individual. For those who learn to use them, the stones become lifelong companions. Like any relationship though, working with stones on an energetic level requires time. It is necessary to take an active interest and build a rapport.

Stones exercise an influence on our bodies by the vibrations they emit, which interact with the electromagnetic field of our body. Elizabeth Beaumont, a gemologist who has an active role in the choice of yoni eggs—their quality and stone—in my online store, explains:

> *The more I learn about the scientific aspect of the mineral world, the more I am fascinated by the intelligence and organizational power of nature. When geological conditions are favorable, crystals are formed that contain the same chemical elements that go into the constitution of human beings, and this confers upon stones an obvious resonance with the human body. Furthermore, in the stones the atoms are arranged in a very geometrical pattern with one another, at very precise distances and angles, exhibiting an intelligence superior to that of a human being, which can aid the human in becoming attuned and in balance with him- or herself.*

It goes without saying that none of these lithotherapeutic properties are intended to replace the advice of a trained medical professional. What I am describing in this book is only an introduction to lithotherapy, which is a vast and inspiring subject. Learning about the power of stones and crystals allows you to realize the beauty of the Earth, your life, and what remains of your journey here. Every individual will have her own path of healing with stones and crystals. It is a path that complements other actions, practices, therapies, and medicines.

"*Practice with stones requires a person to develop their perception. Personally, I have been wearing and using stones for a long time. I have kept them in my pockets, on my desk at school, and now at work or at home. . . . This is a very slow method. It is not a medication that can resolve a health problem in three days; it can take quite a bit of time. It can especially take a lot of time to perceive what is going on inside you and the results that come out.*

Some people think that their worries will suddenly vanish if they stick an egg into their vagina. In my opinion, this practice [works best when it is] performed at the same time as other practices.

MARIE **"**

The best advice I can give you about your choice of stone is to keep listening to your body, your sensibility, and your intuition. The information that follows will give you an overview of the stones used to manufacture yoni eggs, which will help you make a first selection of the ones that "speak" to you most strongly.

HOW TO CHOOSE YOUR STONE

When you first start your adventure in the world of stones, it is not always simple to get your bearings. So I have gathered together here some advice from Elizabeth Beaumont, a graduate of the Gemmological Association of Great Britain and certified by the Montreal School of Gemmology. Elizabeth has offered you some valuable advice on my request.

Through Feeling

We often hear that it is not we who choose the stone, but the stone that chooses us. We are mutually attracted to each other. A person vibrates for one stone. For example, when we pick it up in our hand, we can sense a transfer of energy in our fingers, a tingling sensation, a resonance in our heart, a sensitivity, it can bring tears to our eyes. . . . Several sensations can indicate to us that this stone wants to spend some time with us. This is my favorite way of choosing a stone, because it is a choice made by the heart and not by the mind.

By Color

It is possible, especially when you are just starting out, to associate a colored stone with its corresponding chakra. For example, black, brown, or red stones are connected to the root chakra, while the green or pink stones would be associated with the heart chakra. There is a resonance with the wavelengths of the electromagnetic spectrum of visible light. For example, violet vibrates between 400 and 500 nanometers. Violet stones, like amethyst, will be in tune with the crown chakra, which is desirable for this chakra's balance. At a more advanced level, we are able to contemplate more complex correspondences, beyond the color codes, to obtain the results we want.

For the Properties of the Stones

There are a good number of sites on the internet that offer descriptions of the physical, mental, spiritual, and other properties of stones and crystals. We can often read everything and its complete opposite in this mass of information. How can we get our bearings here? Personally, I favor the authors whose credibility is certain to me. For example, I look to Katrina Raphaell, a pioneer in this domain in the United States, and to Michael Gienger, a mineralogist who performed empirical experiments with his students to discover a common denominator in the properties of stones, in contrast to a lot of other authors who simply cut and paste from one site to another all they find on the internet.

By Chemical Composition

At a more advanced level, a person can select her choice of stone by assessing the chemical components of the stone. For example, lithium is used to adjust individuals prone to mood swings (bipolar personalities). There is lithium in lepidolite, so this stone has calming effects; it helps the individual stay off emotional roller coasters. This is why it helps people recover their inner peace.

YONI EGGS AND THEIR EFFECTS

Here I've listed the optical, physical, and lithotherapeutic properties of the different yoni eggs to help you choose which one is best for you. It is a nonexhaustive list of those I've been able to test for both external and internal use. Of course, this is only an introduction to the information and benefits that these stones can bring to women.

Stones for Internal Use

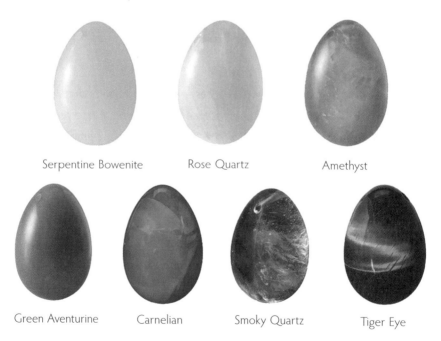

Serpentine Bowenite   Rose Quartz   Amethyst

Green Aventurine   Carnelian   Smoky Quartz   Tiger Eye

Figure 5.2. Stones for internal use

Jadeite
The Traditional Stone

Color: pale green to an intense emerald green, yellow, colorless, white, black, lilac, mauve, red, brown, or blue

Family/group: pyroxene

Crystal system: monoclinic

Transparency: translucent to opaque

Luster: greasy to vitreous

Hardness: 7

Density: 3.3 to 3.36

Benefits: This stone, which is quite prestigious, especially in China, is a symbol of peace and harmony, honesty, serenity, reaching higher consciousness, meditation, and balance.

The jade egg is the egg traditionally used for the yoni egg practice. True jade (jadeite) is very difficult to find and quite expensive.

Nephrite Jade
The Stone of Harmony

Color: often a very deep green but also white, brown, orange, blue-gray, or black

Family/group: amphibole

Crystal system: monoclinic

Transparency: translucent to opaque

Luster: greasy to vitreous

Hardness: 6.5

Density: 2.81 to 3.1

Benefits: Helps find balance of the masculine and feminine energies within, assists with realization, and awakens buried inner knowledge.

The nephrite egg calms and soothes.

Serpentine Bowenite or "New Jade"
The Stone of Protection

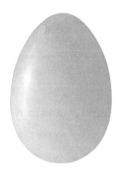

Color: typically yellow-green, but it can also range from solid green to bluish green

Family/group: antigorite

Crystal system: monoclinic

Transparency: translucent

Luster: waxy

Hardness: 5

Density: 2.6

Benefits: This "new jade" offers physical protection from negative emotions and gives us the courage we need to solve problems. It helps us relax, helps us understand our dreams, and is soothing.

The new jade egg is recommended for overcoming stress and moodiness and for finding a balance between the masculine and feminine. It provides a sense of inner peace. Femininity reveals itself. It is a soothing stone of protection that helps us overcome our fears and free ourselves from them.

Rose Quartz
The Stone of Tenderness and Serenity

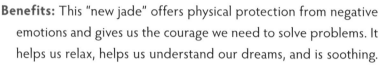

Color: pale pink to bright pink, sometimes with white veins

Family/group: quartz crystal

Crystal system: trigonal

Transparency: translucent to opaque

Luster: vitreous

Hardness: 7

Density: about 2.65

Benefits: It helps establish inner calm, relieves doubts, and steers us toward serenity and self-esteem. This stone reinforces self-confidence and kindness; it heals the wounds that have collected in the heart.

The rose quartz egg is wonderful in encouraging the heart to open as well as kindness, rest, and tenderness, as rose quartz is the stone of love. It helps establish inner calm and serenity, it strengthens love of self and self-esteem, and it helps a woman feel more feminine. It gives hope and relief.

Note: This is a fragile stone that is sensitive to shock and sunlight. By gently taking care of it, you will help take better care of yourself. It can be purified in water.

❝ *I felt the need to get a second yoni egg six months after I had gotten my first one. I studied my options and very quickly the rose quartz made itself known to me for self-confidence, on the one hand, and on the other, for tenderness, soothing, femininity, and so forth. As was the case with my first stone, our duo began working well right away!*

LORIANE ❞

Amethyst

The Stone of Wisdom, Temperance, and Transformation

Color: lilac to deep violet

Family/group: quartz crystal

Crystal system: trigonal

Transparency: transparent

Luster: vitreous

Hardness: 7

Density: about 2.65

Benefits: It supports concentration and mental calm, and it encourages clarity and serenity. It also facilitates good judgment (independent of the ego) and free thought, and it helps us transmute energies and accept reality. It encourages dreams as well as intuition because our more relaxed state of mind allows their subtle messages to be heard.

The amethyst egg brings wisdom and is a source of spirituality, and so it is ideal for meditation, for encouraging deeper sleep during the night, and for awakening the sacred feminine.

Note: Avoid placing an amethyst egg in sunlight or moonlight as it prefers shadow and dark spaces. Amethyst is fairly sensitive to being bumped. When put in contact with other stones, it purifies them.

Green Aventurine or Aventurine Quartz

The Stone of Comfort and Serenity

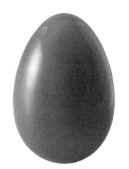

Color: sage green to deep forest green

Family/group: polycrystalline quartz, quartzite

Crystal system: hexagonal

Transparency: transparent to translucent

Luster: vitreous

Hardness: 6

Density: about 2.6

Benefits: Encourages inner tranquillity; cultivates patience and tolerance when you are confronted by situations that normally cause you stress. Allows acceptance and gives you the ability to turn the page on situations that have no way out; it allows you to calmly find your center in yourself while remaining open to others. It supports you in making good choices, choices that are decided in love and not fear. This stone encourages independence and regeneration.

The aventurine egg is ideal for emotional and hypersensitive women, as it will relieve their anxieties and help them recover a sense of lightheartedness. This is a very gentle egg that allows a woman to find emotional and physical balance and to see more clearly the emotional bonds that are preventing her from moving forward.

Note: Aventurine is not especially sensitive to shocks. Some Amerindian rituals use it for reconnecting with the heart. It is purified in water and salt and recharged by sunlight.

Carnelian

The Stone of Joy and Vitality

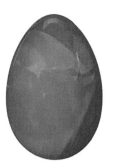

Color: orange to red (due to the presence of iron oxide), sometimes with white stripes

Family/group: polycrystalline quartz, chalcedony

Crystal system: hexagonal

Transparency: translucent to opaque

Luster: vitreous

Hardness: 6 to 7

Density: about 2.6

Benefits: This is a joyful stone that offers vitality and energy. It encourages blossoming, courage, creativity, and relaxation and supports women who wish to have children as well as those who wish inner transformation. It helps relieve emotional disorders and helps people with confusion or overly emotional mental states recover their center. It is also an excellent remedy against sterility and loss of desire.

The carnelian egg encourages the resolution of conflicts and the ability to live in the moment. It helps you find sexual balance and realize the beauty of life. It can be worn between painful periods to help regulate your periods. They will be gentler and of better quality.

Note: This is one of the most beautiful stones for a woman and for couples. It is connected to the second chakra (the energy center at the navel), and it can be placed on the belly for fifteen to twenty minutes during pregnancy and painful periods to soothe them and raise the vibrational rate. It can be purified in salt and water and recharged with sunlight.

Smoky Quartz
The Stone of Rootedness and Stability

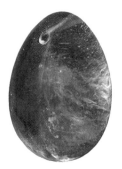

Color: light brown to deep saturated brown, if not black

Family/group: quartz crystal

Crystal system: hexagonal

Transparency: translucent to opaque

Luster: vitreous

Hardness: 7

Density: about 2.65

Benefits: This stone encourages responsibility and getting back on center. It allows you to calm your anxieties and mental or emotional agitations. It facilitates making good decisions, discernment, and balance between light and matter. It allows you to begin a new chapter in life that will be made stable and balanced by establishing sensible boundaries and making your own choices. It dissolves negative energies.

The smoky quartz egg makes it possible to connect with your body and to feel rooted in it. It encourages realization and helps establish a balance between the material and the spiritual.

Note: Smoky quartz calms people who are too "hyper."

Tiger Eye
The Stone of Inner Strength and Physical Anchoring

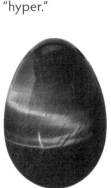

Color: yellow-brown to golden brown, reminiscent of the iris or coat of a tiger, striped by shimmering reflections

Family/group: polycrystalline quartz, metamorphic

Crystal system: hexagonal

Transparency: very slightly translucent and most often opaque

Luster: vitreous

Hardness: 6

Density: about 2.6 to 2.65

Benefits: This stone allows us to see our inner resources by freeing us of certain blocks; it helps us clarify our intentions and find the courage to live them. It is calming and reassuring. It prevents and calms stomachaches and intestinal pains.

The tiger eye egg helps dispel doubts and supplies motivation, and it provides us with the will to achieve our plans by moving past all difficulties. It gives us get-up-and-go and the desire to be in touch with the people close to us.

Note: This is the stone to wear for an exam or an important meeting. It is not terribly sensitive to shocks. It can be purified in salt and water and recharged by sunlight and moonlight.

Quality Stones and Crystals

Some semiprecious stones can be toxic because of the chemical elements they contain, but whether they are safe for internal use usually depends on how they are prepared. Stones like tiger eye, for example, are toxic in their raw form. A raw stone is rough, unpolished, porous, and prone to sloughing off flakes or even microscopic pieces.

In contrast, good-quality yoni eggs, like the ones that are available on my websites (see the resources section at the back of the book), are polished stones that have been selected by gemologists. The polishing is extremely fine due to a sandblasting process. They are perfectly stable and will not deteriorate. It would require temperatures much higher than those of the human body, extreme pressure, or long exposure to certain kinds of radiation (UV, X-ray, gamma ray) to alter their structure.

So there is no contraindication for using yoni eggs made from tiger eyes, unless you plan to crush them into powder and eat them!

Stones for External Use

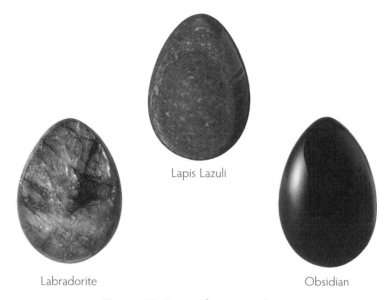

Lapis Lazuli

Labradorite   Obsidian

Figure 5.3. Stones for external use

A number of stones offer fantastic energetic properties but, for reasons of safety, are not recommended to be carried inside the vagina. This is the case, for example, with lapis lazuli, whose small pyrite crystals can flake off inside your vagina.

However, you don't need to deny yourself all the energetic benefits these stones provide; instead, you can work with these stones in meditation or in a crystal lattice.

Remember, the more highly polished your stone is, the less porous it is, thereby reducing the possibility of chemical elements finding their way into your body.

Lapis Lazuli
The Stone of Communciation

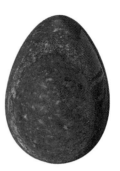

Color: dark night blue, often speckled with white calcite and starred with pyrite so that it displays a golden metallic luster

Composition: rock consisting of lazurite, calcite, sodalite, and pyrite

Transparency: opaque

Luster: vitreous to resinous

Hardness: 5.5

Density: 2.7 to 2.9

Benefits: This stone is helpful for purification. It is also a stone of communication; it allows you to express yourself more freely and clearly, with greater authenticity. It encourages self-confidence, lucidity, intuition, and creativity. This stone will raise your consciousness. It is a purifying agent on both the mental and spiritual planes. It purges karmic residues from the aura. In ancient Egypt it was considered a stone of the gods.

The lapis lazuli egg allows you to express yourself freely. This stone of the gods during the days of ancient Egypt is in fact the stone of communication. While lying down on your back, apply the lapis lazuli over your throat or over your third eye. You can also hold the egg in your hand or keep it in your pocket when you are speaking in public.

Note: When used at night, this stone accelerates dreaming, but its effect can be too intense in the bedroom. It is a fragile stone that is easily scratched and sensitive to shocks, sunlight, and acids. It can be purified in unsalted distilled water and recharged by moonlight.

Labradorite

The Stone of Protection

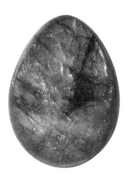

Color: Gray, made iridescent with hints of blue, green, yellow, or orange and more rarely with pinks or violets

Family/group: feldspar, plagioclase

Crystal system: triclinic

Transparency: transparent to opaque

Hardness: 6

Density: 2.65 to 2.75

Benefits: This stone provides protection from negative influences, alleviates mood swings, and stimulates intuition. It is often used by healers and by people who have to meet with many other people over the course of a day. It brings hidden talents to light and helps with the spontaneous expression of our child heart. It is excellent for dissolving illusions.

The labradorite egg, for external use, can be held in the hand for dealing with a case of the blues or a drop in energy, or even when in contact with people whom you feel are negative, toxic, or invasive. It also is of help in finding your life's path.

Note: Labradorite is best used externally on the throat and in the hand. This stone is recommended for use during menopause. It is sensitive to shocks and scratches. It can be discharged in a container full of water during the night and recharged with sunlight.

Obsidian

The Stone of Shadow and Balance

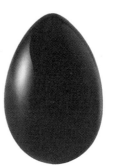

Color: flat or iridescent black, sometimes speckled with white ("snowflake" obsidian)

Family/group: natural, volcanic glass, mineraloid

Crystal system: amorphous

Luster: vitreous

Hardness: 5 to 5.5

Density: about 2.4

Benefits: This volcanic glass dissolves emotional and mental blocks and helps you free yourself from bad behaviors. It is also a stone of protection and balance.

The obsidian egg makes it possible to illuminate zones of darkness and has therefore proved to be excellent for freeing yourself of collected resentments, fears, and anger. It is powerful; it is a question of being ready to confront your own dark side and go deeper into the work. This is not a stone for beginners. Take your time before moving on to obsidian. I only recommend it for external use because of the advanced work and precautions that it requires.

Note: This stone cannot be programmed. It is slightly sensitive to shocks. No purification is necessary, but it loves heat, sunlight, and moonlight.

HOW TO TELL A REAL STONE FROM A FAKE

What our Mother Earth cooks up in her geological kitchen is of superior quality—on the energetic plane—to what is manufactured in a factory or laboratory. Here are a few clues from gemologist Elizabeth Beaumont that will allow you to make your selection of a yoni egg in a knowledgeable way.

When various chemical elements are present together in the ideal geological conditions of pressure and temperature, we witness the birth of a crystal. The atoms assume position in relation to each other with an undeniable geometry at extremely precise distances and angles. Here, the symmetry dictated by the laws of nature is like the stitching of a 3-D sweater. Despite the millions of possible combinations, there are only seven crystal systems: cubic, hexagonal, trigonal, tetragonal, orthorhombic, monoclinic, and triclinic. This organization gives crystals greater thermal conductivity than amorphous substances—that is, those substances whose atoms, or chemical elements, are placed in random fashion (examples: amber, obsidian, manufactured glass, or plastic). Crystalline minerals are therefore cold to the touch (place the stone on the inside of your wrist or over your temple to better feel it), contrary to amorphous substances like plastic or industrial glass, which have a more lukewarm sensation to the touch. You should realize that if you are looking for a piece of obsidian, an opal, moldavite, or amber, you will not be able to distinguish them from artificial materials using this technique, although these substances are natural, given the fact that they are also amorphous.

How can you recognize manufactured glass? Elizabeth tells us that

it is lukewarm or even hot to the touch. If it is transparent, you will be able to see bubbles on the inside, swirls created during the casting, and sometimes bubbles that have been sliced open on the surface, which look like perfectly round craters.

If the material feels very light in your hand when compared to the crystal it is intended to imitate, and it is lukewarm to the touch, then it is probably plastic. If you are not sure, then stick a heated needle into it (in the least visible area, like the piercing hole). It will give off an acrid odor. Amber can be mistaken for plastic, but if you use this test with the heated needle, it will give off a very distinctive and pleasant odor. If this aroma resembles that of pine resin, then what you are testing is copal (the yellow version of amber).

There are many different kinds of imitation gemstones manufactured from non-natural and synthetic products. I hope the advice above will help you be more astute when the time comes to choose your stones.

ELIZABETH BEAUMONT'S ADVICE FOR TAKING CARE OF STONES

Natural stones should be treated with care if you want to keep them in good shape for as long as possible. Here is some valuable advice from Elizabeth Beaumont on this subject. I will give you some of my own personal recommendations for the energetic cleansing of yoni eggs later in the book.

In all cases, you should always opt for natural, unadulterated materials.

The More Fragile Stones

Stones that have a hardness level of five or less on the Mohs' scale are less resistant to being scratched. You should therefore avoid washing them with water or cleansing them with abrasive substances like saltwater because this might remove all their beautiful sparkle. An energy cleansing with sound (using a Tibetan singing bowl, crystal bowl, tuning fork, bell, or so forth) or a suffumigation with sage would be more appropriate.

Discoloration

Many people love to recharge their stones by placing them in the sunlight. You should be aware that the color of some stones will fade over time and become paler and paler. The color may even disappear entirely if they are exposed too often to direct sunlight. This is the case with the family of quartz crystals and colored varieties like amethyst, citrine, smoky quartz, rose quartz, prasiolite, and so on, or even stones from the spodumene family like kunzite and hiddenite.

Temperature Shock

There is a risk that some stones might crack apart if subjected to large deviations in temperature. This is the case with the quartz crystal family; again, that's rose quartz, amethyst, rock crystal, smoky quartz, and so forth. If you want to run them under water, then it is preferable that the water be the same temperature as your stone. Like the stones are to the touch, the water should be colder than the ambient temperature. You can then gradually add warm water so that the overall temperature of the water increases very gradually.

Flaws

Some stones have fault lines, which is to say that in some direction the electrons are not bonded together as strongly. If the stone suffers an impact in that direction, it will split in half. You should therefore be mindful of the impacts that your stones might be vulnerable to and never allow them to fall onto a hard surface. This is the case, among others, for fluorite, topaz with calcite, diamond, feldspar (moonstone, amazonite, sunstone, labradorite), selenite, and scapolite.

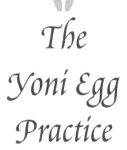

PART THREE

· · · · · · · · · · · · · · · ·

The
Yoni Egg
Practice

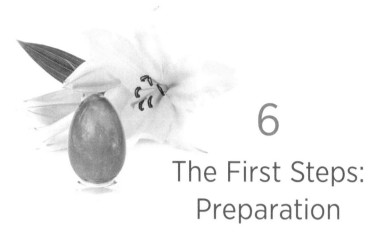

6

The First Steps: Preparation

If this is your first time using a yoni egg, you may feel apprehensive and have some concerns. You are probably questioning yourself, your body, and how you will start the practice. You nearly feel ready to take the plunge, but not quite. You might be afraid, and that is perfectly normal. You do not need to rush into it; the right moment to begin the yoni egg practice will come to you when the time is just right.

GETTING TO KNOW YOUR EGG

The first thing you need to do is get acquainted with your egg as if it were a new friend. A "hello" to get started would be nice. There are as many ways to get familiar with your egg as there are women in the world. For some women the right time is right away, while for others it will first be necessary to establish a relationship, and still other women will want to wait until just the right moment.

Women Who Are Impatient

66 *I was in a hurry to try my egg, yet I waited for three days to get used to it. In the beginning I walked around with it in my purse.*

SOPHIE 99

66 *I did not take a lot of time before using it. Just enough time for introductions and an exchange. . . . Tonight will be our fourth date.* 99

STÉPHANE

Women Who Are Patient

66 *I took the time I needed to get acquainted with my egg. I slid it under my pillow and slept with it for several nights in a row. I also held it in my hand and caressed it for several days straight. I think I put it inside one month after I got it, when I felt the right time had come.* 99

LAURE

66 *I did not put my egg inside me on the first day. I waited. Today, I sleep with all my eggs, and I put one inside once it has decided. It sounds bizarre, but that is just how it happens.* 99

BÉATRICE

66 *I have a large egg made of rose quartz because I had four children. It took me two or three weeks before I could begin using it. I slept with it under my pillow, and then, one afternoon when I was alone, I tried it out as an experiment. It went in ice cold and came out nice and hot!* 99

MAUD

66 *Since I began the practice, I have had one surprise after another. I took a long time getting to know my eggs, but since then I feel like I've come back to life. I have become the person I used to be again: sweet, funny, full of enthusiasm and compassion . . .* 99

MURIEL

Advice from Users

A lot of you have given me your advice for encouraging other women. Here are the main things:

- Take your time.
- Listen to yourself.
- Trust in yourself and in your instincts.
- Try out the egg for a brief time, and then try it for longer periods.
- Tame it little by little.
- Go gently, and use a yoni egg that has been pierced and has a string through it, especially for the first few times; this helps avoid needless panic and makes it easier to remove the egg.
- Wait for just the right moment, wait for the desire to be there, wait for the moment when you are ready to be open to new possibilities
- Become friends with your stone before ever using it.

" For the first time you use it, you should not get tense and stiff. It is better to breathe, relax, and use coconut, sesame, or almond oil. "
EMMA

" You should not look for any kind of result but just observe how your body reacts to the egg while you caress your body. It is extremely important to detach yourself from the image of a woman masturbating. You should not make yourself feel guilt for savoring a female moment. It is like a moment of meditation. "
MARIANNE

" The first time, I remained lying down. I did not keep it in for very long. I felt it would be a good idea to listen to myself and gently insert it. When my yoni is ready for this, it opens. You have to gently remove the egg when you have had enough; it is as simple as that. "
FLORENCE

PREPARING YOUR YONI EGG FOR THE PRACTICE

✢ *Clean It Physically*

Before using your yoni egg, clean it. Everyone will have their own method for preparing the egg, but you have to be very disciplined about keeping it clean.

Carefully wash your egg with gentle soap or a vinegar solution, then rinse it, beginning with water that is the same temperature as your stone and gradually increasing the temperature until it reaches lukewarm. Then dry the stone with a clean, dry towel.

If you have chosen an egg with a hole pierced through it, blow into it, or you can clean out the inside of the hole with a small interdental wire brush. This will require a little more time.

Mantak Chia recommends steeping "the egg in water that has had tea tree essential oil added to it. The wire of the brush should be replaced each time it is used. Rinse well."

Osteopath Corinne Léger also appreciates the use of tea tree essential oil: "It has antiseptic and antifungal properties (against fungal infections like athlete's foot), as well as antiviral properties. It is also recommended for dealing with problems caused by parasites (like *Trichomonas vaginalis*). This essential oil also has anti-inflammatory, antioxidant, and healing properties. It possesses a large spectrum of activity yet remains harmless to vaginal flora and the mucous membrane."

> ❝ I used Aleppo soap to clean my egg before and after using it. I applied authentic lavender essential oil to it beforehand and tea tree essential oil to it after I used it.
>
> AURÉLIE ❞

To avoid any needless worries, remember that we do not sterilize or scour clean the penises of our men or our fingers before penetration or contact with our vaginas! Similarly, we can be satisfied using whatever hygienic measures seem appropriate to us for the egg.

✣ *Clean It Energetically*

Looking at it on the energetic plane, your yoni egg is going to enter into contact with you and with the energies that are enclosed inside your yoni. All the stones have energetic properties that they can transmit to you, but your yoni egg is also going to absorb and cleanse the negative energies that have been lying stagnant inside your yoni. For your egg to retain its "energetic punch," it must be regularly cleansed of the bad energies that it picks up from us. Later in the book I will share with you some valuable tips for performing this energetic cleansing—during rituals—with creativity and intuition.

✣ *Program the Egg*

Before putting the egg inside, set your intention to engaging with this part of your body to hear what it has to tell you and to allow it to guide you. In part 4 of this book, I will explain in detail about the power of intention and the way to put your intention out there to program your yoni egg.

✣ *Anchor the Egg*

Some yoni eggs are pierced with a hole so that a string can be attached to them. The string will allow you to pull the egg back out when you wish to do so. This will help give you the reassurance you need during your initial experiences with the egg to become familiar with it, the practice, and your yoni.

I have a definite preference for yoni eggs that have been pierced horizontally through the smaller end of the egg, though some are pierced vertically. It is the largest part of the egg that is inserted first, which means that the string that is attached to your egg will end up extending downward, like the string of a tampon, making it possible to easily pull out the egg.

Find a cotton string (like the kind of kitchen twine used for trussing a roast), a piece of dental floss that has not been waxed or mentholated (the most natural one you can find), or a fishing line (this is less pleasant to wear, however). My preference is for cotton string, even though it is easier to thread the yoni egg with dental floss.

Once you have found your string, cut a length that is equal in length to the distance between your elbow and your hand. Then fold it in half.

Thread the hole in the yoni egg with the folded piece of string, then loop it, then make a knot at the end of the string (see figure 6.1). You are now ready to use your egg!

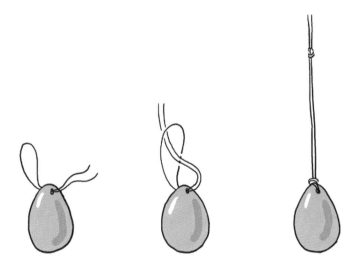

Figure 6.1. Threading your yoni egg

PREPARING YOUR BODY FOR THE PRACTICE

✦ Making Your Yoni Smile from the Inside

The practice of the inner smile, as taught by Mantak Chia, is a simple and valuable tool for accompanying the practice of the yoni egg. He explains:

The practice of the Inner Smile begins in the eyes. They are linked to the autonomic nervous system, which regulates the action of the organs and the glands. The eyes are the first to receive emotional signals and cause the organs and glands to accelerate at times of stress or danger (the fight-or-flight reaction) and to slow down when a crisis has passed. Ideally, the eyes maintain a calm and balanced level of response. Therefore, by simply releasing your eyes, you can relax your whole body and thus free your energy for the activity at hand.*

Allow the feeling of relaxation to spread throughout your entire face, your skull, your bones, and your body. While you breathe, maintain a smile in your consciousness. Naturally, a smile will appear on your face.

Inhale and exhale deeply while smiling. Your breathing will become filled with greater joy. Now direct your smile toward each of your organs. Send it downward like a trickle of water through your jaw and neck, then through your lungs to the liver, the gallbladder, the pancreas, the stomach, and the spleen on the left. Next send it to the kidneys, in the center of the lower back, without forgetting to focus on the adrenal glands, the bladder, and then the stomach, the intestines, the colon, the sexual organs, and your yoni! Direct your smiling energy toward your yoni. It will become filled with energy. Take a moment to visualize this energy full of life spread throughout this part of your body: the vagina, uterus, fallopian tubes, ovaries, clitoris, labia, and so forth. Continue smiling as you feel this internal massage, and savor every minute of it.

Maintain this inner smile all throughout your yoni egg practice and, if you wish, until the end of the day.

Aisha spells it out more explicitly, as follows:

---

*From *The Inner Smile: Increasing Chi through the Cultivation of Joy,* by Mantak Chia (Rochester, Vt.: Destiny Books, 2005, 2008), 26–27.

Quite simply, the fact of spending time smiling in your yoni may appear a bit strange, but it is truly the foundational practice of the jade egg. It is the means of becoming aware of this space. Allow the yoni's energy to embrace the entire space of the vulva, the space of the vagina, the outer and inner labia, and all the internal openings; this is known as the jade cavern. It is the key that opens a gate; you enter into the cavern and next into the jade palace! This palace is where your goddess dwells. It is a very sacred and beautiful space.

❖ Self-Massages for Releasing Blocked Sexual Energy

Before you make any use of your yoni egg, it is recommended that you put yourself in a state of joy with the help of several forms of self-massage. These are not masturbatory practices but actually energetic and emotional preparations to ensure that your work with the egg takes place in the best possible conditions.

Here are a couple of examples suggested by experts in this domain.

◈ Sarina's Recommendations: Cat Paws Self-Massage

This exercise was described by Sarina Stone during one of my interviews at the Tao Garden Health Spa and Resort in Thailand. It is the result of her years of practice and studies guided by Mantak Chia.

The cat paws technique is quite simple. Cats perform this kneading movement with their paws when they want to stretch or simply try to make a sleeping spot softer. I invite you to do the same thing by practicing these delicate gestures. Place your hands flat over your stomach. Apply a gentle, alternating pressure with the palms of your hands, and then your fingers, on both sides of the stomach. If a particular spot seems painful, then press on this part of your body with your fingertips, while breathing and smiling, until it becomes limber again. When you are done, wait a minute or two for the energy to circulate again, not forgetting to smile at your organs while doing this. You can visualize yourself like butter that is becoming soft.

◆ Shashi's Recommendations:
 Yoni Massage to Release Emotions

Our yoni stores all kinds of memories. I found the advice of tantric expert Shashi Solluna, whom I interviewed on the island of Koh Phangan in Thailand, extremely insightful for preparing for the insertion of the egg.

> *I like to recommend that the woman begin by lightly pressing on the different parts of her yoni opening with the egg and then letting it rest there for a certain amount of time. Small contractions might be felt; this is the yoni beginning to vibrate and then relax. Very often this produces a feeling of intense emotional liberation. Many tears may spill, but this is a good thing. This makes it possible to open the contracted spots on the yoni. You can then continue to massage your yoni with the egg.*
>
> *During your first times, take a lot of time to massage yourself, and particularly to massage your breasts, while keeping the egg placed at the opening of your yoni. Imagine that the opening to your yoni is like the hands on the face of a watch. Press lightly on the opening of your yoni while traveling along the clock face. Hold the pressure for several seconds at each spot, and breathe. You hold, you breathe.*

If you begin your yoni egg practice by massaging yourself, your yoni will be ready to receive the egg and to communicate with you. It is a magnificent gift to offer to yourself.

The yoni is a very deep and secret space that can store memories that, once they have been brought back to your awareness by the egg, can trigger strong emotions and tears. Don't be surprised if your yoni recovers its youth, its spark, and its confidence and if it becomes more limber after this liberation! It is a process of self-healing.

✤ Lubrication, If Needed

If you have the sensation or conviction that you are not wet or lubricated enough before inserting your yoni egg, take a little more time to get yourself into that condition.

Rub your hands vigorously together. Bring your heart energy into them and start by massaging your belly and then the insides of your thighs, the bone structure surrounding your genital organs, and your yoni.

Feel the heat and the love energy that is starting to open up and causing the tensions in your entire body to dissolve. Breathe. Smile and place one hand over your heart and the other one over your yoni. Say the sound "hawwww" three times and smile.

Cause your arousal to rise, caress your breasts, caress yourself, or use coconut oil. You can also use aloe vera; this plant has wonderful healing properties for any hurt or irritation inside your yoni. Furthermore, it refreshes naturally.

> **❝** I particularly like to use coconut oil for massaging myself, and I like to smear a few drops of sandalwood essential oil on my yoni egg.
>
> BENÉDICTE **❞**

Don't hesitate to use a natural and organic oil (such as coconut oil) to help provide better external hydration of your intimate areas; this will facilitate the introduction of the egg. Wearing your egg inside yourself and practicing the rituals and exercises described in this book will help the vagina to better create natural lubrication later.

Relax and appreciate this personal moment to take care of

yourself, to massage yourself, and to prepare yourself for the yoni egg practice.

"" *When I feel the desire and when it's okay, I choose the right stone based on the day. I strip myself nude in a room with subdued lighting, and I slide the cold egg on the opening of my vagina. I hold it there with one hand while I caress my breasts with the other. I can feel the energy that is awakening in me, and I can feel my egg that is gently sucking it in.*

MARIANNE ""

KEEPING A PERSONAL JOURNAL OR LOGBOOK

Keeping a personal journal or logbook will help you make greater progress in your practice. In it, you can note your observations, emotions, fears, actions, and discoveries, as well as the kind of egg you used, what size it was, when you used it, and even your realizations that arise from this practice. You will be able to jot down what is working for you, what is not working for you, and what you are learning about yourself. This will help you gain confidence as you practice. Keeping a personal journal is one of the elements that will allow you, after you have worn the egg, to build your confidence over time and establish a personal connection with your yoni.

You should write down in your logbook the hour, date, place, and duration of your practice, as well as the kind of stone you used and the size of the egg. You should also note what you felt, what you observed, and even what you may have revealed about yourself. Pay attention to the signals your body is giving you, to the information it is giving you, and to all the things you feel that you are releasing inside. See the box on pages 105–6 for a sample of what your logbook might look like.

When you vary the type of stone, the size, the weight, and the practice, new sensations will appear. Your sensitivity will increase over time, and this personal journal will become a treasure trove of information.

Personal Journal or Logbook

This personal journal or logbook will allow you to gather together all your notes on your yoni egg practices and rituals. You can use the logbook to write down your feelings, your observations, and what you learn about yourself and your body.

The outline below shows what you might want to include in your logbook on first learning about the practices of the yoni egg, on discovering *your* yoni egg, and impressions of subsequent rituals and practices with your egg or eggs.

Discovering the Yoni Egg

Begin by writing down revelations, *aha* moments, and advice that has resonated from your reading of this book, including the passages that were most illuminating for you and the personal stories that touched you most deeply.

My First Time

Date and time:

Place:

Size of the egg:

Gemstone of the egg:

Pierced or not pierced:

Duration of the practice:

What I felt and observed:

What I learned:

My before/after:

My Practice

Date and time:

Place:

My intention:

My practice of the day:

Size of the egg:

Gemstone of the egg:

Pierced or not pierced:

Duration of the practice:

What I felt and observed:

What I learned:

What I am grateful for:

What advice my yoni gave me:

My personal notes:

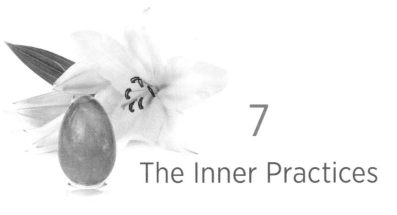

7

The Inner Practices

INTRODUCING THE EGG INTO
YOUR YONI FOR THE FIRST TIME

You are now feeling ready to welcome your egg inside you. Your yoni is feeling increasingly enthusiastic about the idea of this new encounter and exciting discovery.

Lara Castro, sexologist and yoni egg expert, makes the following suggestion.

> I encourage you to feel the texture of your yoni with your hand before inserting the yoni egg. Learn to recognize yourself. We are better able to detect what is going on in our bodies than anyone else. Use a mirror to look at this part of your body. Keep watching while you spread open the lips of your yoni and touch it inside.

It is quite natural if you feel shy on this very first time. This encounter and exploration can be made more comfortable with the following recommendations. I therefore suggest that you read this book entirely before beginning your egg practice. With the knowledge here, accompanied by your growing desire to put it to use, you will be ready and enthusiastic.

✣ Insert It Gently

Begin by finding and creating a private space in which you can carry out your yoni egg practice. Ideally, you will be all alone in the house.

> " I use it when I am alone in my room, and I take the
> instructions from the book into consideration.
> I caress myself; I smile . . . It is exquisite.
>
> RACHEL "

After you have washed your hands and your egg (in accordance with the hygienic conditions that would apply when you are inserting any object inside yourself—and which are explained in the preceding chapter), heat the egg either with your hands or by running it under lukewarm water (the stone is often a little bit cold at the start but pleasant this way to some women). If you like, put on some relaxing music and light a candle to help you unwind a little and prepare yourself for the practice.

The practice can be performed while you are standing up, seated, or lying down. Pick up the egg with your left hand and place it over your heart. Place your right hand over your yoni.

Say the "hawww" sound three times. Feel the love, joy, and warmth of your heart in your whole body and in every single cell. Take a deep breath. Focus your attention on your genital organs, observe them, and ask their permission to perform the practice.

If you get an answer of "no," don't proceed. Feeling a "no" means that you are having doubts or fears about the practice. It also implies that your body is not ready at this moment. Don't judge yourself; simply observe and respect this temporary "no" from your body. It is normal to feel apprehensive the first time. Take a breath and wait for a better time, whether that's later on the same day or on another day. When you are ready, you will feel comfortable and excited at the thought of starting off on your new adventure. In the meantime, continue spending time with your egg and asking your yoni to let you know when the right moment has arrived.

If you feel that you are ready, place your egg in contact with your yoni. To support this encounter, position it gently against your labia majora and slowly make circles with the egg over them until it finds a comfortable position. Breathe deeply and slowly. Using the inner smile technique, bring your heart's love energy down and take some more deep and slow abdominal breaths. José Toirán suggests introducing "your yoni egg into your yoni while in a positive mental state, accompanied by an inner smile and an outer smile."

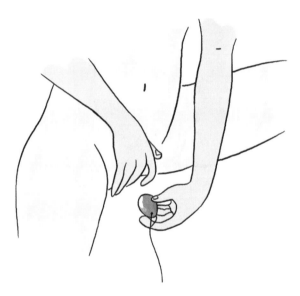

Figure 7.1. Preparing to insert your yoni egg

Free your thoughts by feeling the contact of the egg on this part of your body. Feel its temperature and gentleness. Breathe deeply and gently until the moment feels right. As you inhale, feel your yoni "sucking in" the egg, and feel your vagina opening with each exhalation, as if it were yawning. It can take some time to actually feel this. Breathe, and visualize the insertion of the egg taking place without any problem. The larger half of the egg will go in first, with the smaller end through which the string has been threaded last.

Once you have placed your yoni egg close to your vagina, it will more or less be sucked in from the entry point. How strongly it is sucked in depends on your muscle tone. Help push it inside with your finger but without forcing it, just like you would insert a tampon. Your yoni egg will find its place in your vagina and stay warm there!

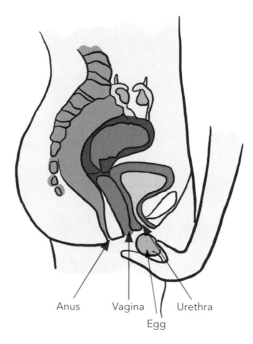

Anus   Vagina   Urethra
Egg

Figure 7.2. Inserting your yoni egg

If your egg will not stay inside you, it is possible that it is not the right size. If this is the case, try using a larger yoni egg. If the larger yoni egg does not stay inside, your yoni needs physical training (which will be described later in this book), or a visit to your gynecologist is in order for a more extensive examination of your pelvic floor.

❝ *I stuck it in all at once without any fear. It was no more complicated than putting in a tampon!*

VALERIE ❞

> *" I immediately liked the contact with this egg, which I had patiently inserted without any difficulty, and with a real pleasure (something entirely new for me).*
>
> ISABELLE *"*

❖ Keeping the Egg Inside You

Once you have inserted the egg inside your vagina, the first step is to learn how to keep it inside without losing it. Mantak Chia explains how.

You are practicing with the yoni egg just by wearing it, even if at the beginning the egg falls out or does not stay in place because of the muscle tone of your perineum. No need to panic: if you wear underwear (not too tight), it will catch the egg. Clean it, reinsert it, then resume what you were doing.

He continues:

Learning to keep the egg inside without losing it is a good first step of the process. The key is learning how to keep it inside yourself, after which you can walk about your house. If you are worried, you can contract your vagina and train yourself to make the egg stay in place.

José Toirán shared this tip with me: if you are worried about losing the egg, tie the string of the egg to your underpants!

It is possible that your egg will slip out when you go to sit on the toilet, when you are hysterically laughing with a friend, or when you sneeze. Your uterus moves in such situations, and that can push the egg toward the outside. With a little training, you will remember to contract your muscles and bring the egg back up into the middle of your vagina. You can even play with this squeezing motion to cause the egg to move up and down. These contractions will help you achieve greater mastery over your egg.

Don't be overly expectant in the beginning. Allow your body and your yoni to act at their own speed. Just let go. Entertain yourself, alone or with your partner. Your body will interact with the egg, your sensations will progress of their own accord, and they will increase your connection and your understanding of your yoni. Move.

> 66 *It is true that I began to feel my whole yoni better,*
> *and because I was able to contract it during sex, I felt a*
> *more intense orgasm. I feel like a beautiful journey*
> *has started, and I am going to stick with it.*
> CLARE 99

✤ Take Breaks

It is vital to note that the time you take to rest between practice sessions is just as important as the time you dedicate to the exercises provided in this book. During this resting period, you can observe your yoni, listening for its messages and supporting the changes it is undergoing that will allow it to rebuild itself.

It is not recommended—especially when you first start following this practice—that you keep your yoni egg inside you for an entire day. Listen to your body and pay attention to the sensitivity of your yoni, which will now start expressing its desires more and more clearly. Several minutes of contracting and relaxing the muscles of your vagina should be enough at the beginning.

If you have used your yoni egg for an entire day, then a rest of one or more days is recommended. As I will explain to you in the next chapter, you can perform specific exercises with your yoni egg, or you can just simply have it inside you for several hours during the day, while squeezing and relaxing your muscles around it from time to time.

Jutta Kellenberger confirms the value of approaching this practice based on feeling.

> *You can do it every day if you like. It is not necessary to do it for*
> *a long time; several minutes should be enough with a concentrated*

practice in which you focus on yourself. The nervous system—in other words, the mind's activity—should descend into the vagina to reconnect with it. You concentrate so that you can feel when you contract around the egg.

⚜ How to Remove Your Egg

Getting your yoni egg back out is not always so sexy. Sometimes you have to proceed based on the moods of your egg and your yoni. I am teasing a little here, but sometimes we really do get the feeling that our yoni does not want to have the egg inside her . . . and she knows how to tell us that! Perhaps you will suddenly have the sensation that you need to go to the bathroom for a number two, for example.

Though it's probably not necessary, it's worth saying up front that from time to time the yoni egg will put us in the embarrassing situation of having to find it and then fish it out of the toilet bowl. Yes, this is a reality that will most certainly accompany our practice! It has some surprises in store for us, especially at the beginning!

If you have the feeling that the egg wants to stay warm where it is, perhaps it wants you to work with it a little longer. If it wants to stay where it is for a more extended period of time, as long as it is neither irritating nor painful and you are feeling calm, leave it where it is and listen to your yoni.

If you want to pull your egg out, take a deep breath, then exhale while gently tugging on the string. Relax; it will come out!

> ❛❛ *I trust in my ability to contract and expel the egg if I want to do so. I am already quite happy that my egg stays inside me for as long as I want and that I can manage to expel it by myself.*
> NATHALIE ❜❜

If you do not have a string and you would like to get the egg out quickly, simply cough, laugh, and push and it will come out. If that doesn't work, squat down and lay your egg. Don't panic! It will eventually come out. One time, I kept mine in for six days! That's not something I would recommend, but when I was first starting, thinking I was clever, I put the egg in without a string. The egg made the decision to stay snug and warm! Now, thanks to practice, I can push it out whenever I wish.

> ❝ *I had a large egg that did not have a string. After twenty-seven hours of panic, because I could not reach it, it came out on its own naturally. Since that day I know that the egg can push itself out on its own.*
>
> ELIANE ❞

> ❝ *I have an egg that I adore. I am not scared that it will stay stuck inside me because I trust my body. I love it, and I have always found it courageous and connected.*
>
> VERONIQUE ❞

BEGINNING THE PRACTICE

You made it, you are here, and you are ready to begin your yoni egg practice. Here are several exercises to get you started. You can perform them in almost any position: lying down, seated, kneeling, or standing up.

As you just learned, when the time comes to put the egg inside, let out a sound, or a sigh if necessary, and then bring the egg in contact with the entrance of your yoni. Insert the egg as described above. Moving gently, slightly undulate your body. Allow the egg to make its way in gradually and very gently.

Once the yoni egg is inside you, continue breathing and sending the egg onward by contracting and relaxing your vaginal muscles to build up your muscle tone. Add a gentle movement of the pelvis. If you like, you can squeeze more strongly when inhaling, pulling the egg inward, and then push the egg outward when you exhale. In this way, the egg will move from the outside in and vice versa. You can accompany this exercise with a slight swaying of the pelvis if you like.

José Toirán explains:

When you are doing your practice with the yoni egg, observe your body (your neck, your shoulders, your tensions). Relax, observe yourself again, and give thanks. Then take intentional actions based on this. The yoni egg can often make you aware of a problem in the body that deserves attention. It makes taking proactive action possible.

As you are moving the egg within you, focus your awareness on the egg's presence in your body. The sensations will become more and more perceptible with regular practice. Observe the sensations in your body and, afterward, note down in your logbook (see pages 104–6 for more on creating and keeping a logbook or personal journal) what you felt during the practice or ritual you performed. Also note what you liked about the practice and anything else you observed.

When you are first beginning the yoni egg practices, you may not feel the egg at all. That's normal. Your sensitivity will increase over time. Your focus, in the beginning, should be directed toward understanding and observing the difference between relaxing and contracting. There will be no shortage of emotions that arise during this process. "Many emotions are contained in our yonis. With the practice of the yoni egg, some of these emotions are going to be released," sexologist, psychotherapist, and yoni egg expert Lara Castro reminds us.

When your body and your yoni feel ready, try to push the egg to expel it.

"If a woman finds it easier to expel the egg than to make it rise inside of her, that is often a sign that she gives a lot to others, to her family. She will gain much by working with her egg, granting herself some moments that are just for her, to find her own space," explains José Toirán.

Here again, it will not be easy in the beginning, but it will become so in a very short while. The string can help you pull out the egg, so don't hesitate to make use of it. Personally, I do not use the string very much because now I have trust in my egg and I can make it come out whenever I want. I know my body better, and I find that it is able to expel the egg easily on its own. If you have difficulty, review some of the options described above (see page 113).

> 66 I place my egg in front of me like a treasure, and I smile—
> in my body and on my face. I massage my belly while
> breathing, I listen to my body and give it thanks, and I introduce
> my egg to my yoni with some delicate assistance. I try to visualize
> it rising and descending in rhythm with my
> breathing—that's the stage where I am at this moment.
> I always keep it in for a few hours afterward until I feel
> that it wants to come out.
>
> CÉCILE 99

SETTING OFF TO DISCOVER YOURSELF

Following are a few exercises given to me by Mantak Chia that I would now like to share with you. Between each of the exercises, energize your hands by rubbing them together, massage your belly and the area over your ovaries, and then raise your hands to your heart and massage your breasts in all directions while focusing on creating more compassion and beautiful energies. Remember to perform the inner smile and to smile on the outside too. A positive and joyful state of mind is important for the yoni egg exercises.

✣ Exercises to Strengthen the Organs

Lie down, then breathe in and press/squeeze your yoni egg into your vagina. Inhaling, raise your pubis as high as possible. Exhaling, relax and return to the ground vertebra by vertebra. While doing this, make "mmmm," "oooh," or "aahhh" sounds (opening the throat is important; this is something that will develop over the course of your practice).

◈ Moving the Feet in Alternation

Stretch one foot forward, maintaining awareness that this movement originates inside the genital organs. Your hips should be relaxed and able to move freely. Take your time. Place your hands over your lower belly and bring your awareness deep into this area. Return your foot to the starting position. Repeat with your other foot. Alternately stretch each foot, focusing on its connection to your lower belly.

◈ The Windshield Wipers

Spread your legs open slightly and simultaneously point each foot inward. Keep your feet flexed like this for the entire exercise. Bring your feet outward by clenching your buttocks, then swing them inward until your big toes are touching. Repeat. Feel how the genital organs are working on the back-and-forth movement.

Important

Take a break between each series of exercises. Keep your tongue relaxed and in contact with your palate. Smile at your body. If you feel any kind of discomfort, massage the region with your loving hands and rest. Do not continue. You are in the process of making your muscles work, and they can become tired or painful in the beginning.

✤ Exercise of the Three Orifices

During a workshop that we organized for her and José Toirán in Bordeaux (France), sexologist Lara Castro offered the following exercise, which I find worth sharing with you.

In your logbook, write down what you feel and observe at each of the stages of this exercise. The realizations that arise about your body, your yoni, your emotions, and your sensations are valuable clues for improving your practice, gaining a better understanding of your own body, and continuing to make progress. All this will help you to fully enjoy the benefits and secrets of the yoni egg.

1. Place the egg inside your vagina, hold on to the string, and make a series of contractions and relaxations of the yoni.
2. Focus on the three orifices: (1) your urethra, (2) your vagina, and (3) your anus (see figure 7.2 on page 110). Close each of them separately in the order of 1, 2, 3 and then 3, 2, 1. What are you feeling? Can you identify these three orifices? If not, turn back to the discussion of anatomy in chapter 1 and review that material, while using a mirror, because it is essential to know these parts of the body to practice the yoni egg exercises.
3. Learn to distinguish between the upper and lower triangles of your yoni by first contracting the vagina and urethra together, followed by the anus. This is the upper triangle. Then contract the anus and vagina together, followed by the urethra. This is the lower triangle. Note which of these two triangles contracts most easily for you.
4. Visualize the ischium bones (the curved bones that form the pelvis; they support the weight of the body when you are sitting down) and try to push as if to make these two bones touch. Anatomically this is totally impossible, but the point of the exercise is to look for a sensation. Ask yourself, "If I were able to do this, which muscles would I have to contract?" Close your eyes and identify what is moving inside of you. Find the best position for doing this.

   Next, imagine that your coccyx and pelvis are coming into contact with each other. Identify the movement that would make this happen. Then combine the two movements—bringing the ischium bones together, and bringing the coccyx and pelvis together—alternating between one and the other; don't forget to breathe.

   Finally, try to contract everything at the same time. Count the number of seconds that the contraction lasts, and rest, with all your muscles released, for twice as long as you had them contracted. (This rule holds true for all the exercises performed with the egg.)
5. Adopt the position of a cat: get on all fours, then round your back

and arch up. This position allows you to relax your pelvis. Notice whether the egg moves.

6. Sit down with your buttocks on your heels, then stretch out your arms, your back, and your entire body.

7. Gently take out your yoni egg and take a moment for yourself in peace and quiet.

✢ Advanced Practice

This last technique is more advanced, and it is one of those that has been introduced by Mantak Chia. It is for women who have an established yoni egg practice. These women can add little weights to help make their yoni work a little harder. This is something you can try after you have practiced the above exercises regularly for several weeks or months. This is not a technique that everyone can practice. Listen to what your body and feelings are telling you.

For this exercise, you'll need a little pouch with a cord. If you buy an egg from my website, it will come with a pouch, or you can look for something similar.

Once you have put the yoni egg inside, take a deep breath, contract, and cause the egg to move. Put several jewels, gemstones, or crystals inside the pouch to give it weight. Then tie the string of the pouch to the string of your yoni egg. Standing with your legs spread and the pouch with the small weights between them, squeeze your yoni egg and force it to move. This practice will improve the muscle tone of your vagina, and you can gradually increase the weight. If the weight is too heavy for you, your vagina will not be able to keep hold of the egg. If this is the case, reduce the weight and try increasing it over time.

I would like to repeat: the goal is not to have a "super muscular" yoni but rather to give it the power to release its full power and pleasure and recover its muscle tone. Be attuned to what your body tells you.

It is better to use a jade egg or one made from aventurine for this advanced practice because these stones are more solid and resistant than others, especially the quartz stones.

A Practice for Men

Men can also use jade eggs. They will not use them for the same reasons or the same benefits, nor in the same orifice!

Mantak Chia recommends the use of a small egg for men. "It is necessary for men to choose a jade egg of the smallest size. It is absolutely essential that it have a string attached to it. Lubricate your anus and insert the egg little by little. To feel the egg, you will have to squeeze the muscles of this region. Then cause the egg to move up and down with the help of the string."

José Toirán adds: "It is essential that a string is attached to the egg because, contrary to the case when it is inserted into a vagina, the egg can move deeper inside the body. Start by bringing the egg close to your anus and playing with it before inserting it. The G-spot for me is in the anus. Not only will this give your prostate a massage, but it will also allow you to feel great pleasure."

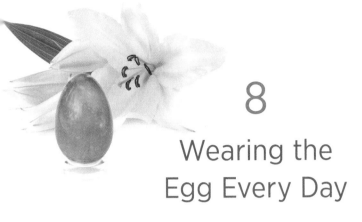

8
Wearing the Egg Every Day

There are many different ways to use your egg in your daily life as an active woman. You can also use it alone or with a partner. Taking some time for yourself every day by secretly holding the egg inside you is stimulating and exciting! It will allow you to be radiant in even the most trivial everyday situations.

> " *I experimented on how safely I could wear the egg by just keeping it next to my sex for a long time, neither inside nor outside. I just kept it in personal contact without any impatience or force. This gave me a sense of security in my womanly integrity.*
>
> BENÉDICTE "

> " *Since I began using the egg, I've been more aware of my vaginal muscles and my internal movements. My G-spot has recovered its sensitivity, and my uterus has relaxed. I no longer have any menstrual pains, nor any pains when snuggling. I don't have lower backaches anymore.*
>
> LUCIE "

" *As soon as I pick it up in my hand I feel as if I am filled with an infinitely sweet and powerful energy, and I have not let it out of my sight for two days (I keep it in my hand). In the beginning I used it at home, then I began to carry it when going out and going to work. I still hardly ever put it in; on the other hand, I am almost never without it. Its contact with the palm of my hand, or its presence in my pocket or my purse, gives me a sense of calm and security.*

SIDONIE "

WHAT'S THE BEST PACE?

When you feel that you are fully familiar with the egg and its practices, you can intensify your work with it. You just need to respect several rules of hygiene and stay in tune with your body. Always listen to its messages and remove the egg when you feel discomfort.

" *I use it several times a week, depending on how I am feeling.*

EVELYNE "

" *I cannot practice more than twice a week. I can only use it when I am not working because I cannot wear the egg during periods of stress like at work. I prefer to do it at times that are respectful of my natural rhythm.*

MIREILLE "

" *I connect with myself, and I feel or squeeze the egg to develop my muscles. I use it around five days a month, no more.*

ALICE "

" *I don't use it on any regular basis. I feel when I'm ready to receive one. When it's okay, I choose the appropriate stone and I stretch out to perform some contraction and relaxing exercises. Then I keep the egg in for around one hour.*

CHLOÉ "

PAY ATTENTION
TO YOUR FEELINGS

To use the egg, you must truly feel ready from within, with your heart, body, and yoni all on the same wavelength. During the time you are doing the yoni egg practice, stay tuned in to your feelings. You must take the egg out if you feel any discomfort, itching, irritation, or inflammation or if you experience any vaginal discharge. Discharge could indicate a fungal infection caused by a change to the vaginal flora. In any case, do not force yourself to put the egg in or keep it in, as this is not the purpose of the practice. Simply listen to yourself and, most importantly, give yourself time.

WHEN AND WHERE

At Home

In the Daytime

We all have a thousand domestic activities on our to-do list: laundry, tidying the kitchen, doing the dishes, and so forth. Take advantage of these times to wear your yoni egg. If you are scared of losing your egg while you are out of the house—at work, for example, or while you are walking down the street—practice at home: put on some music at home, insert your yoni egg, and start dancing! This will be both reassuring and effective. If you dare, strip off your clothes and stroll around the house naked with your egg, whether in silence or with a little music. If you have a partner who returns home a little earlier than anticipated, he or she will likely fully see what has changed in you! It is not something that a partner will find displeasing . . .

> 66 At home I have time and I can get comfortable. I wear
> my egg for several hours. Sometimes I go out with it in,
> and I've sometimes even done yoga with it in.
> DIANE 99

> " *The practice that intuitively inspired me was to 'wear'
> the egg every day, like an accompaniment. I cannot practice more
> than twice a week, and I wear it only when I am not working
> (the weekend and Wednesdays), because it doesn't work
> for me during stressful times like those I experience at work.
> I need a time that matches my natural rhythm.*
>
> SOPHIE "

At Night

If you are an experienced practitioner and you do not have any specific worries, then you can wear the yoni egg all night long if you feel the need. This period of serenity during slumber is extremely favorable for establishing a good connection with your yoni. Allow yourself to be cradled by this singular contact and sleep in complete peacefulness.

It is not recommended, however, that you wear the egg for several days or nights in a row. Listen to your body and to the messages your yoni sends you.

Osteopath Corinne Léger states, "There is no risk in sleeping with a yoni egg. You might choose the rose quartz for its very soothing properties, qualities that encourage deeper sleep and better recuperation."

> " *For the moment, I only use it at night because
> I lose it too quickly during the day. I put it in
> in the evening before I go to bed.*
>
> CÉCILE "

In the Bath

A bath offers a wonderful time for relaxing and connecting with your femininity. It is also a golden opportunity for using your egg and practicing with it while you are relaxed.

My Tip

I love to light some candles, put on some relaxing music, and add some essential oils and three or four handfuls of unrefined coarse sea salt to the bathwater to help me relax, put aside my worries, and find myself again. I also take the opportunity to submerge my yoni eggs in the warm water, and I insert a small yoni egg so I can do my exercises in the bath. I like to add several of my yoni eggs into the bath to clear their energies with the salted water. It also infuses the water of my bath with great energy.

✤ Ecstatic Bathing

Minke de Vos, an expert Taoist instructor, has created and teaches a large number of ritual practices to be performed in water. Below is one that I find particularly delectable: "ecstatic bathing."

Put some essential oils and even some flowers into your normal bath. Wear your yoni egg. Let yourself be carried by the water; let your hair float around you. Pull on the string of your egg as if you were tugging a boat through the water, and your entire spinal column will move like a serpent. The kundalini energy rises. Relax your neck, your nape, and your head, and this will release all your tensions. When you are in a state of relaxation, your natural energy begins circulating in a very beautiful way all through your body. You will adore this! It is a magnificent form of practice.

You can invite your partner into the bath. Let yourself go completely by suggesting that your partner pull gently on the string of your egg. Your yoni will naturally let the suction pull it in. I call this "travel love." It brings to mind a gentle game of tug-of-war, in which two opposing teams pull on opposite ends of a rope. Allowing yourself to be guided in this way makes it possible to achieve a wonderful state of relaxation. Stop thinking about anything except your sensations.

In the Evening after a Long Day at Work

The end of the day is a great time for wearing your egg. When you are feeling exhausted but you have not had a chance to wind down, even though you are now at home, the egg is a good way to make a complete break with your hectic day, as well as any external demands, and just get back to yourself.

> " I realized that I often got easily annoyed in the evening. So I got into the habit of putting out the intention of spending a peaceful evening and inserting my egg before seven o'clock. This is how I manage my exhaustion at the end of the day.
> ÉMELINE "

In the Bedroom

If you are in a relationship, you may decide to tell your partner about your practice. Of course, you can also decide to keep it a secret, something that is just for you, but sharing it during foreplay can turn both of you on. Some women like using the egg during sexual relations. Rose quartz is a perfect stone for this practice. Because it is subdued and delicate, it will know just how to accompany you. If your partner is open and curious, experiment with the yoni egg together to discover new sensations and unheard of pleasures!

You can also use it by yourself, of course.

> " I use it when I am alone. I go into my room, I caress myself, I smile . . . It's exquisite! I also use it during the day to strengthen my pelvic muscles and to give me energy.
> RACHEL "

At Work

"You can wear your egg at work, and the egg will work for you all day long," José Toirán told me during a live interview he gave me at a Paris theater in September 2015. But, he mischievously added:

Don't forget to wear some underpants! Everything will be going along just fine up to the moment when you start laughing, and at that moment the uterus will begin ejecting the egg. . . . This happened to one of my students during the middle of a coffee break at work. But she was quite clever—she exclaimed that the pocket of her skirt had come unstitched and, without anybody noticing, she grabbed the egg and put it in her pocket.

This got a huge laugh from the audience.

Wearing your egg at work is both simple and effective. During your morning routine, after you have showered, simply insert the egg into your vagina and presto, head off to work. During meetings or when you are in front of the computer, say a little hello to your egg by squeezing it and then relaxing. Even if you forget it is there, it will still keep working in you. You can wear it for several hours in a row; your yoni will be working simply by holding it inside.

Shashi Solluna explains the benefits you can draw from wearing the egg during the day.

All day long, while in front of our computer, we can take advantage of it to tighten our yoni back up as well as to make our energy rise again. This can reprogram our entire body in very short order. People do this every day, and the energy rises back up. The invitation to make the energy rise instead of letting it remain stuck in the sexual core puts the body into a state of orgasmic ecstasy.

She goes on to say:

When you start causing your energy to rise up your body like a wave, you become vitalized and relaxed. With experience, you can feel it rise like a fountain throughout your entire body.

❝ *I got a promotion at my job, and when I have important meetings during which I know I will have to assert myself, I wear it. I feel calmer, focused, and poised.*

Eᴠᴇ ❞

❝ *There was a man at work who spent his time silently staring at me, judging me, and being jealous of me. By wearing my egg, I felt more like a woman, and the fear I had of this man vanished.*

Sᴏʟᴀɴɢᴇ ❞

Tips for Work

If a boss, coworker, or client is being particularly difficult, think of the egg you are wearing inside. This should help you not take the situation too much to heart and to remain centered in your good-will bubble. Feel that you are being supported and accompanied from within!

You could also take advantage of your lunch break to wear your egg and/or perform some small contraction exercises while you are eating. If you are in the habit of leaving work to exercise during your lunch break (going to the gym or yoga studio, for example), remember to put your egg in your gym bag, and do not forget to include your cleaning solution too. You may decide to wear the egg while you are exercising, staying mindful of contracting your vagina to keep the egg inside you while you are performing certain exercises and to increase its presence and effect.

During a Date

If you have fallen for someone and wish to gain more confidence for a date together, I highly recommend that you wear your egg! You will be the only person to know that you have it inside you. You will feel at the top of your game, and this will make you even more irresistible. Wearing the egg will let you support your energy and observe how being with this person manifests your heart's desire within you. If this is not your first date together, then take note of any changes that have appeared in your date, as well as in yourself, since you started wearing the egg. Even if you have known this person for quite some time, you should still pay attention to any changes. You should also observe and note how people behave toward you in your everyday life.

Precautions for Wearing the Egg in Public

If you wish to wear your egg in public, you should be aware that there are some circumstances, places, and situations in which it would be better for you not to wear it. To begin, there are some things to keep in mind concerning your anatomy: if you cough, laugh, or sneeze, your egg can suddenly find itself on the ground, depending on the muscle tone of your vagina and the energy that is circulating at the time this event takes place.

If your yoni egg should happen to fall to the ground, following is some advice for dealing with the situation elegantly. You can discreetly pick it up without anybody seeing. You can claim that there is a hole in your pocket and it allowed an object to fall out. You can tell whoever is around that you will tell them more about it later. If you are with a romantic partner, you can tell him or her that it is a kind of surprise. Or you can just say, "oops," and simply pick it up.

Following is a list of situations in which you really need to pay attention to holding in your yoni egg:

If you have a cold (you're likely to sneeze or cough)

If you are working out or otherwise exercising (exertion can cause an egg to fall out)

If you go out dancing (you're likely to be active)

If you are going to the bathroom (you may inadvertently release the egg)

If you are not wearing any undergarments (which would allow an escaped egg to fall freely)

PART FOUR

Revealing
and Liberating
Your Sacred
Feminine

9

Initiating Yourself into the Power of Your Egg and Your Yoni

Do not expect to immediately receive the full range of potential benefits as soon as you start using your egg. You will start to feel changes within a short period of time by observing the days you practice and the days you do not. Most of all you will need time to build a relationship with your egg in order for it to bring you what you are expecting of it. Avoid building up too many expectations! Don't imagine that your egg is going to solve all your problems! What it *will quickly* do is shed light on the inner work you need to pursue. In fact, the yoni egg alerts women to their need, for example, to get started on a program of personal fulfillment, or to begin physiotherapy, or to consult a gynecologist about a pain that has been crying out for treatment over a period of time. It offers revelation on every level! You just need to stay attentive.

The same holds true for life. *If we expect to experience some beautiful adventures, and we can feel them coming and are ready to welcome them, our mind-set encourages happy events.* But having unreasonable expectations does not always allow you to appreciate all of life's surprises. Write down in your personal journal what you discover, over the course of your practice, about your body, your yoni, your needs, your stones, and so on.

❝ *Just go with your natural rhythm! You need to be curious and expect nothing; that's when you will have surprises!*

ALIX ❞

Listen to Your Intuition

Listen to your intuition, for it will guide you! Whether it concerns the size of the stone, the kind of stone, the way you should wear your egg, or even the time of day when you should do the practice, it is a valuable tool for getting in tune with your body and your inner wisdom, and getting into harmony with both.

Every woman knows her own body—or will learn to know it. Intuition will allow you to go beyond appearances, and sometimes even logic. Teach yourself to listen to that gentle voice that offers you guidance. This inner wisdom will become more and more present on the outside.

Be Creative

If you are feeling apprehensive in anyway, take your time. Never force the egg to go inside. Practice with your yoni egg during a time of joy, and give your desires as well as your creativity free rein.

Not all of us are ready to introduce the egg into our yoni, and even for those of us who have practiced for a while, on some days the yoni says "no." Because the egg is a powerful symbol, if the yoni is not ready, you can simply carry the egg in your hand, or in your purse. In fact, I recommend that eggs made from certain stones, like labradorite, lapis lazuli, or even obsidian, be used only externally. Holding them in your hand allows you to build self-confidence, to gain a sense of inner security, and to dare to say things in a genuine and truthful manner.

To each her own yoni, and to each her own yoni egg practice! Give free rein to your creativity!*

To Each Her Own Rhythm

We all have a different way of practicing that is based on our body, our health, our age, our stress level, and our daily life. There is no specific rhythm that we need to impose upon ourselves. Regular and frequent practice is essential, but so are periods for rest and relaxation. It is often said that it is more important to relax than to try to accelerate your rehabilitation by overdoing it. You will only do yourself a disservice by overexercising this part of your body. So, again, listen to what your yoni has to tell you and find your own personal rhythm.

Begin by performing a ritual for introducing your egg to your yoni, then make a date with yourself several days later for putting it inside your vagina. But make sure that your yoni is amenable. Perhaps in the beginning you will want to wear it only for twenty minutes while you are at home to familiarize yourself with it. Whatever you decide, know that there is no hard-and-fast schedule for yoni egg practice, and every woman will have to discover her own rhythm.

The Egg Is Part of a Greater Whole

Working with the egg is only one stage and one tool among many others in a woman's life. It will open the doors of knowledge and curiosity, which will allow you to procure new forms of contentment and new pleasures. In no case is it a final point or period for your development, nor is it an answer to all your worries as a woman. Don't mistake your egg for a magic wand! For most women, however, using the yoni egg opens a magical door to liberating traumas, insecurities, and guilt they may have been storing for a long time. It opens them to new therapies, fresh advice, and most of all tapping into

_____

*I encourage you to share your experience and recommendations with other women and friends on my private English facebook group, Lilou Yoni Eggs, https://m.facebook.com/groups/666758977112978?ref=share.

their inner wisdom instead of relying only on outside sources and expertise.

Use Your Egg Regularly

Like any practice, without regular and dedicated time using the egg, it will not be able to provide positive and lasting results. Buying an egg and simply being satisfied to stare at it will not solve your problems with incontinence! Stepping into an unknown new practice will enable you to explore new possibilities that you can't yet foresee. It is an exploration that you need to do with openness, gentleness, and regularity.

> 66 I bought my yoni egg in 2017. It has been enthroned ever since on the top of the dresser in my room. I have not used it yet; however, it is there every day.
>
> GENEVIÈVE 99

Women who do not get any results are very often the same women who have only used it once, or at best use it very rarely (once a month at most). (Other reasons for a lack of results could include prolapse of the pelvic organs or a serious personal health concern that requires professional treatment. The yoni egg can be quite helpful after such problems have been treated as an adjunct to physiotherapy and follow-up care.)

Whatever her personal situation, body, and history, every woman will be able to find her own rhythm, determine how to use the egg, and develop her creativity, intuition, and attentiveness. We are all unique, ladies, and so are our yonis!

PROGRAMMING YOUR EGG

The power of intention has been described and used for a very long time. It has been almost twenty years—the time of my first steps on the path of personal development—since I took an interest in this inner power and wisdom that we all possess and that I can feel bubbling inside me.

I wanted to learn from the best teachers: Wayne Dyer, Jack Canfield, Tony Robbins, Don Miguel Ruiz, Caroline Myss, Paulo Coelho, Bruce Lipton, Gregg Braden, Louise Hay, Dan Millman, James Redfield, Sonia Choquette, Joe Dispenza, and hundreds of others around the world. I spent the past twelve years interviewing them, watching their videos, and reading their books.

They made it possible for me to realize that my outside life is a reflection of my inner world. I then began transforming my life, on a day-by-day basis, by learning to receive and listen to my inner wisdom. But what I found to be most effective, which I applied in the program I cofounded in 2005 with Sandy Grayson and Laura Duksta—the 100 Day Reality Challenge—is the power that comes from setting an intention every morning.

The idea that we can co-create our life every day rather than suffer through it inspires me, and it pushed me to move forward, drawing unprecedented events into my life. Since then, my life has become more and more thrilling, one step at a time, because I've made myself an active participant in it. I love knowing that I am able to collaborate in the co-creation of my life (way beyond direct action and knowledge). I no longer need someone to bring it to me on a silver platter. I know that I am responsible for my life and can make it as great as I wish through my own transformation and the power of vulnerability and authenticity. I no longer want to lie to myself or accuse the system or others for my bad days. We are delicious co-creators!

If I think that life is unfair, then I will attract unfair situations that will prove to me that I am right. If I wish to attract a new companion, then I am going to start feeling gratitude now for making his acquaintance in the very near future. The situations and challenges I am going to meet on my path will help me grow by learning eternal soul lessons. My intentions will gain greater clarity; my happiness won't be conditioned by outside circumstances.

Little by little I allowed myself to be who I really am. Today I lead a life that befits me, in which my creativity, my energy, my enthusiasm, my skills, and my talents are all in the service of something greater.

The yoni egg is receptive to intentions and sensitive to frequencies as well as vibrations. You have the ability to deprogram and reprogram it however you wish. Try it for yourself!

✧ Clean Your Egg with Energy

The first stage of any ritual with your yoni egg consists of energetically cleansing and purifying your egg of any past programming it might have acquired in its travels, making its way to you. You can read about the rituals for energetically cleansing the egg beginning on page 156. You might, for example, choose to leave your egg for two or three hours in direct sunlight, or you might cleanse it using sage. You can also use the power of intention and invocations to ask for your egg to be purified. The most simple way to purify your egg is to place it under running water in your sink and ask the water to wash away memories that could have been stored in your yoni egg.

✧ Define Your Intention

Once your egg is purified, start writing down your intentions in your personal journal or logbook or on a piece of paper. For example, you might write, "I want to be free to be myself," "I want to have confidence in myself," "I want to free my sexual energy," "I want to connect to the goddess within," and so forth. After you have drawn up this list, identify the intention that speaks to you most strongly right now.

Your intention should seem extraordinary to you but feel possible. Clearly state your intention in writing in the form of an affirmation: "I am freely making my choices. I assert them in love and complete serenity. I feel good and full of energy."

✧ Infuse Your Egg with Your Intention

In a calm and pleasant environment, pick up your egg with one hand and hold it over your heart. Place your other hand over it. Forge a connection between your egg and your heart. Feel the stone coming into coherence with your heart. Think of your intention—if you need to, take your journal or the piece of paper on which it is written—in the form of an affirmation, and repeat it several times. Feel the joy and emotion of living that intention from this moment forward. Connect with your heart to amplify this intention. Give thanks, breathe, and smile. Visualize and feel the infusion of your intention into your egg.

✤ Keep an Eye Out
for Signs and Synchronicities

After you have formulated your intention and therefore "programmed" your yoni egg, start your practice. Insert it and wear it so it gets into resonnance with your own magnetic field. Become attentive to the signs around you. Be ready to observe and tune in, and then act as your intuition tells you. Your sixth sense is innate and natural. All it asks is to be heard. But do not forget to keep striving and trying. Our intuition often presents to us a piece of information, a danger, or an opportunity in the form of an image, a message, or an impulse that may sometimes seem illogical.

As your intention takes hold in your life, synchronicities will occur in greater number and offer opportunities for transformation and change. They are all quite simply a magical rendezvous with life: You find yourself at the right spot at the right time or, in other words, facing a situation to which your intellect alone could never have led you. You may find yourself drawn to a piece of information, an object, an individual, or an event that you could never have imagined or been able to foresee. And yet it holds great significance and quite often leads you to make a decision, a realization, or a transformation.

If you decide to wear your egg for several hours during the course of the day and you find yourself having negative thoughts, remind yourself that it is there; squeeze it with your yoni by performing several contractions and releases. It is connected to your intention.

LEARN TO COMMUNICATE
WITH YOUR YONI

Many of us are disconnected from our yoni. We don't have to look very far to see how we behave so as to attract the attention of someone we are interested in, to be loved, or to feel desirable. When we are disconnected from our yoni, we are also disconnected from our innate mysterious and creative power.

Our yoni has much to tell us and sends us extremely clear signals. But the fact is, too often we wait until we are suffering—from an infection or a leaky bladder, a painful or burning sensation, worries about getting pregnant, or a loss of libido—before we finally start listening to this part of our body. However, our yoni reflects our moods and our state of mind. It cannot lie to us. It is a valuable ally.

Discovering the voice of our yoni takes us far beyond the advice that we can read or hear. It knows what is good for it—and for us. Rediscovering this communication will contribute to a greater love and respect that you grant yourself. You will then be in a position to make better choices, from partners and sexual practices to self-expression, which will play a huge role in giving meaning to your daily life.

✤ Give Your Yoni a Nickname

If you have never connected with your body in this way, and specifically with your yoni, then this exercise might make you uncomfortable. So have fun with it as it will allow you not only to establish contact but also to communicate more subtly with your yoni and co-create with her!

Lie down or sit in a place that is quiet and where you will be left alone. Breathe slowly for several breaths. Place one hand over your yoni and one hand over your heart. While continuing to breathe slowly, bring awareness and presence to this part of your body. Once you feel that your heart rate has slowed and you feel you have made a connection with your yoni, ask it what nickname it would like to have: Sacred Flower, Orgasmic Cave, Blue Lotus, Feather . . . Feel its response and then agreement when it likes one of these names.

Repeat its name several times softly and aloud, tell it hello, and thank it.

✤ Invite Your Yoni to Speak

When you feel ready, indicate to your yoni that you would like to receive its wisdom, and invite it to speak or communicate with you.

You can facilitate this communication by writing the message you feel emanating from your yoni in your personal journal or on a piece of paper: "I, [your yoni's nickname], would like to tell you that [the message your yoni has to give you]." It might have past memories to clear out with you or emotions, fears, or wishes to express. For example, you might write, "I have felt ignored and betrayed by you recently. I have noticed that . . . I would like it if . . . It would be helpful if . . ." Allow yourself to write freely without judging yourself for five to ten minutes. Allow whatever is coming out to be on paper. Then read and notice what resonates true and important to you. Then take actions accordingly. Your yoni might need to feel and hear your love and respect for her from now on. She will open herself up as you encourage her from a place of love to liberate her voice and advice.

If you feel an imbalance, ask your yoni, "What can I do to restore balance?" If you want to have a child but are experiencing difficulty in getting pregnant, tell it, "I would like to be a mother. Do you have any recommendations?" If you have met someone whom you would like to get to know better, ask your yoni, "What do you think of this person?" If you would like to meet someone special, ask your yoni to guide you toward the love of your life. The idea here is to communicate in complete simplicity to reinstall trust and intimacy and to reforge a connection.

Ask your yoni your question, listen to its answer, then act.

You can do this exercise before and/or after your yoni egg practice. Your dialogue will become more and more natural and unforced and will quickly turn quite intimate, as if you were reuniting with an old friend whom you have just found again after many years.

❖ *Thank Your Yoni*

Conclude this exercise by thanking your yoni, with endearments and sweet words, and take action based on the answers it gave you and how they resonated for you. Take the time to communicate regularly with your yoni, be grateful for her conscious presence now in your life, for revealing your sacred feminine, and for this relationship growing and guiding you. You may also find yourself wanting to please her with a massage, having a bath, and making offerings to her. The goddess within you, tuning in to your yoni, will appreciate and give back.

10

Experiencing the Sacred Feminine through Rituals

EMBODYING THE SACRED FEMININE

Countless women have been accused, condemned, or criticized because their ideas, their power, and everything they represented caused others to be alarmed. However, empowering and honoring the feminine principle (not just the woman) is the purpose of the sacred feminine. It does not require that we ignore, push aside, or reject the male principle; instead, it welcomes both aspects in each of us—man and woman. It unifies. It represents the union of the feminine and the masculine, the yin and the yang.

The spirit of men and women is expressed differently through the feminine principle. It does not dismiss the masculine but proposes coexisting with it. One is not better than the other. Both together form a dance, one that makes it possible to find a balance between the visible and the invisible worlds, the inner and the outer worlds, the material and the spiritual worlds, while respecting the nourishing Earth on which we reside and thanks to which our lives are possible.

Gaining Access to the Sacred Feminine in Your Everyday Life

Expressing your emotions opens an access to the sacred feminine. Because emotions are often devalued in society, not all of them should be shown. Sometimes we are scared of them. Accept them for what they are, without judging them or trying to understand them. Be kind when you are confronted by them and by what you are going through. Give yourself the love and compassion that a mother offers her child.

Regard your emotions as a source of important wisdom and information. Our sensitivity offers us enormous access to numerous extrasensory powers that will allow us to make contact with a wisdom that is much deeper and more connected to the world and energies around us. By honoring your own emotions and those of others, you will receive a great deal of information that can guide you and transform certain situations.

Listen to Your Intuition and Act Accordingly

Intuition, or our "sixth sense," is what allows us to know something without knowing how we know it. Thanks to our intuition, we are able to detect dangers and opportunities, and we can figure out people even before reading their profile online or turning to a psychic for information!

To hear her intuition, a woman must learn to trust in and act based on a simple, clear voice that guides her step by step. Without being able to explain it, she will be led into an exciting unknown future. One she cannot predict and one where possibilities beyond her current understanding coexist. This is both exciting and revitalizing: listening to your intuition amounts to co-creating your life in the most sacred sense of the term.

When we listen to our intuition and act upon it, we build our confidence and faith in life itself. As Sonia Choquette, international intuition expert with whom I co-wrote *Le défi des 100 jours! Cahier d'exercices pour developper votre intuition* [The 100 Day Challenge! A book of exercises for developing your intuition], said, intuition allows you to travel at the speed of love. That will knock your socks off; I guarantee it! As you work with your intuition, its signal becomes stronger and stronger, like a muscle that develops once you begin to give it training. Information can come to you quickly and naturally. You can then make quick decisions that are aligned with your heart and soul. Play the "I wonder if . . ." game, as Sonia suggests, to question yourself regularly about your day: "Hey, I wonder if my sacred feminine will help me discover some new quality within myself today . . ."

By listening to your heart, you will enjoy a life that is designed for you, that has meaning, and in which your sacred feminine will guide you to the goddess you are. This will allow you to experience situations in which your soul can act in complete freedom and, therefore, where magic happens! The more you listen to your intuition and act accordingly, the better guidance it will give you. It is a splendid muscle to exercise along with your yoni.

Listen to Your Body's Wisdom

Your body is by far the tool that brings you the greatest details and information about a situation, a place, a person, or an event. It is essential that you listen to your body so you can follow your intuition and let your sacred feminine guide you. The yoni egg, yoga, meditation, tai chi, energy massages, sound bathing, and women's circles, among other things, will help guide you in the development of your sensitivity and ability to listen to your own body. Knowing how to do this will allow you to make choices that are meaningful for you. This marvelous compass consists of the inner truth you can feel inside through sensations like shudders, goosebumps, and so on.

Spend Your Time in Silence

Remember to set aside some time in your overloaded schedule for some moments of silence, meditation, and stillness to encourage contact with your sacred feminine. Gaining access to your inner wisdom, which is connected to life's grandeur and a universal wisdom, involves taking some time for yourself.

Some of your quiet moments will appear completely devoid of any meaning for you, while others will seem to be instilled with grace, new ideas for contributing to the world, new steps for living your life's mission, and ideas for manifesting your version of the sacred feminine.

Connect with Nature

Go barefoot for a while to feel contact with the ground, the Earth. For the same reason, hug a tree, work in a garden, watch the ocean, and connect with the elements and with the rhythm of the Earth, listening to its murmurs and welcoming its wisdom as well as its timeless quality.

Create Your Rituals

Rituals allow us to connect with life force to something that is greater than the self. It helps us experience unforgettable symbolic and magical moments that take place beyond the logical and the visible.

The common denominator of all rituals is that they awaken the sacred, build faith in life, and open us to and make us one with the extraordinary. A ritual gives us the opportunity to be out of space and time, slow down, and connect to universal force and our inner wisdom, ready to serve. It is a privileged moment of meeting your soul, the life force in which you can feel yourself penetrated by life and source. Your mind shuts down, and you are led into dancing with life.

You have no need for a middleman here; you need no priest, imam, or rabbi to experience a direct connection with the source of life.[*] Although such an idea may seem intimidating to some people, you should know that rituals will permit you to resituate your inner power where it should be—within—by reappropriating a space and a time that you have given away to others.

There can be no rituals without intention, without symbolism,

---

[*]Lilou Macé, *J'ai pas de religion et ça me plaît* [I have no religion and I like it] (Paris: Éditions Tredaniel, 2014).

without presence, and without gratitude. Rituals require that you take your place, proclaim your inner power, and open yourself to life's mystery in complete humility. They invite you to go beyond what you already know about yourself and about life, to be a goddess and allow the soul to act.

You can begin practicing rituals at home; all you need is a space that holds objects that are symbolic for you and a room in which you feel good and which will be charged with your energy. You can also create an ephemeral ritual space in a totally natural setting (forest, beach, clearing, mountain), in your garden, near a tree, or even in an unusual place that calls to you and "vibrates" strongly to you.

A ritual can begin with the creation of an intention (this will form the context of your ritual; for example, "My intention is to honor my sacred feminine") and the preparation of what you intuitively feel would be helpful to have available for the ritual (candles, incense, essential oils, yoni egg, stone, poem, gentle music, and so forth).

The next thing to decide is your choice of a place, the people who will be present (that is, whether you perform the ritual alone, as a couple, or as a group) and the time you will allot for it to take place.

After you have opened the ritual with some gestures and/or some words (for example, lighting a candle and stating your intention as "I open the space of the ritual with the intention of . . ."), you may wish to invite the guidance of a benevolent dimension beyond the visible. Then you can perform the ritual of your choice. Let your inspiration of the moment take over. Let yourself be guided by contracting your yoni, your inner creative power, and the goddess that you are. Give yourself permission to honor her and listen to her by way of your heart.

A gesture of acknowledgment and gratitude, such as the "yoni mudra," can bring your ritual to a close (see figure 10.1 on the facing page). The yoni mudra is a hand position practiced to balance the body and connect with your yoni, bringing strength and power. It is practice to honor the woman, who is the creator of life and source of life. Benefits include connecting to the Earth, connecting with the female energy, encouraging balance, supporting women during challenging

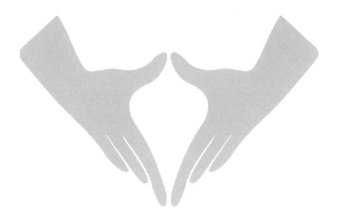

Figure 10.1. The yoni mudra

times, balancing the right and left hemispheres of the brain, and supporting you in making a deeper connection with life.

Over time, you will become more and more at ease with the idea of creating your own rituals. Asking life and the Earth for permission to perform your rituals would be a good habit to cultivate. Find your own words and gestures to express your inner beauty, and the sacred feminine will liberate you and reactivate memories of a past life, allowing you to gain confidence and to restore your inner power to your current life.

With practice, you will be able to discover your own path and your own rhythm. Dare to speak, sing, and dance freely to celebrate and honor life. In this way, you will help transform your body into an instrument. You will be able to allow yourself to be penetrated by this life force more and more naturally, not only during your rituals but also in your everyday life. This is also possible on a collective level. When I interviewed her in Bali, the singer and priestess Suzanne Sterling told me:

> It is important for us to become our own spiritual authority. It is essential that we reestablish public rituals in our society. We are made to express ourselves and live as a community. Finding our truth and verbalizing it in community allows us to discover our path. This is no longer a matter of tradition. The time has come

*to give back in this new age. Many people appropriate things
but do not give anything back. They take but do not give back.
Here, I am talking about giving back to the Earth and also the
community.*

✤ Dance Ritual

Take advantage of a time when you find yourself alone to enjoy a more
subdued light (for example, by lighting several candles) and let your
body dance to some pleasant and lively music that will give you the
desire to free the goddess within you! Do this with the intention of
freeing yourself from the memories of your family bloodline, to open
yourself, to feel joy, and to establish contact with your sacred feminine. Do not forget to ask your yoni to express itself in the dance!

✤ Pacification Ritual

This ritual can give you help during a delicate or difficult moment in
your life. Your intention here is to find relief for this situation.

Settle yourself comfortably on a cushion or in a chair. If you have a
favorite essential oil, breathe in its perfume and allow its aroma to carry
you away, and remain in the space of your heart for several moments.
Next, place a drop of essential oil on your heart and its chakra, in the
center of your chest. I like geranium essential oil as it helps open all the
space around the heart. It supports the opening of the heart in a more
subtle way than rose essential oils, for example. To some hearts, depending on traumas and past experiences, a stronger oil such as rose should
not be the first choice.

Allow the situation that you wish to calm down to rise to the
surface. As you do this, you may feel anger or sorrow rise up. Allow
this feeling to express itself. Give yourself permission to externalize
your emotions. Thank them. Emotions have been stuck in there for
a long time. Don't judge yourself for what comes up, simply receive
and experience the release. A new you will be emerging out of this
experience.

Breathe in and then exhale while connecting with your yoni, connecting with its power and the creative potency that is inside you and that you would like to receive. Recharge yourself with this energy, as if you were a battery.

Holding your hand over your heart, thank yourself for this moment. How are you feeling? Do you have new ideas and new intuitions that you would like to turn to your advantage? If the answer is yes, then feel free to act in kindness and with complete confidence.

WOMEN'S RITUALS WITH THE YONI EGG

It is recommended that the yoni practice be ritualized to make it a wonderful experience outside of our everyday lives—a moment that is magical and unique.

To begin, create a warm, intimate, gentle, and feminine ambience, which will encourage the awakening of your own sacred feminine. Your body will relax, your mind will open, things will become more fluid, and magic will take over, bringing you to a place where you can experience unique moments of connection to your sacred feminine.

For example, light a candle, dim the lights, slip between some silk sheets, immerse yourself in a saltwater bath that has had rose essence added to it, or purify your hands in a bowl of water filled with rose petals before each practice.

✤ Ritual for the First Contact

Take your time during your first contact with your yoni egg. Acquaint yourself with it, contemplate it in the light, feel its temperature and its texture, allow your curiosity to grow, and anticipate what you are going to discover with it.

Your egg has not come into your life by chance. A complicity and intimacy will come into being and fall into place between you. Quite often, when you hold a yoni egg in your hand for the first time, something happens: you feel wonder, surprise, embarrassment, and/or anticipation.

To give the egg a warm welcome into your life as a woman, envision and create a ritual of your choice. Here's an example.

Choose a space and a time that is just for you. Sit on the ground and place in front of or around you a variety of sacred objects, such as fragrances, oils, feathers, drawings, photos, statues, a bowl of lukewarm water (with flower petals in it), and a clean cloth. These are all objects that for you symbolically represent femininity, the sacred feminine, your life as a woman, and the yoni egg.

Begin by expressing the intention of wishing your yoni egg a warm welcome ("My intention is to wish you welcome into my life as a woman . . .").

Next, clean and purify your yoni egg. Thank it for having come into your life and ask it to guide you, to accompany you as well as to support you in your quest for fulfillment and personal well-being.

Now give free rein to your imagination to continue this ritual just the way you would like it to be. At this stage, some women will be ready to insert their egg and experience their first inner contact with it.

When you are ready, conclude your ritual by thanking life and your egg for this first experience.

✤ Ritual Bath

Taking a ritual bath before doing my yoni egg practice remains one of my favorite rituals.

Run your bath and add some rose petals to the water. Light a candle and put on some relaxing music. Create an ambience that will be conducive to relaxation and sensuality. I like to add coarse sea salt to the bath, along with a few drops of essential oil. We will all have our own techniques for promoting total relaxation. Before getting in your bath, gather your yoni egg(s) and warm it gradually under water. Remember to prepare the egg(s) for the change in temperature by only gradually increasing the heat of the water. Then dive in with your egg(s).

Take advantage of this moment alone with your egg(s) to put it into contact with the various parts of your body, including your yoni.

You can massage your yoni with the egg by placing it on your labia. Put some pressure into this massage to release some of the energies that are stored there. This is a time to get acquainted.

✤ Purifying Your Hands

Before starting any practice, it is a good idea to purify your hands. There are several ways to do this. You might, for example, simply let water from the faucet flow through your fingers, or, more symbolically, you can plunge your hands into a bowl of lukewarm water (enlivened with some rose petals, if you wish). Feel the water on your hands and running through your fingers, and place your awareness in this part of your body. Feel the sacred feminine that dwells inside of you, and thank life for this moment. Then dry your hands with a clean towel and light a candle.

✤ Ritual of the Letter

Find a comfortable place to settle in with pen and paper. Write a letter to your yoni expressing love, reconciliation, or forgiveness. Begin it by writing, "Dear Yoni . . ." Set a timer for ten minutes and transcribe, without stopping, all your thoughts. Give yourself permission to write down your secrets, your regrets, and your frustrations; free your memories and your emotions in an attitude of understanding and kindness. Mention what your yoni egg practice and your new relationship with your yoni are going to bring you. Truthfully write down what you want.

Keep your letter someplace safe, bury it, or burn it. Choose the ritual that suits you best so that you feel free and relieved with regard to your past relationship with your yoni. This symbolic act will free some past energies and emotions that are impacting your present, the NOW, since you are placing your attention on it. If you want to create a bright future for yourself and unleash the goddess within, the letter will contribute a step among many along the way to total freedom. It is powerful to stand for what you want. You are affirming the new you to emerge and live new possibilities.

❖ Ritual for Dreaming Effectively

Before going to bed, light a candle. Lie down. Feel your body on the bed; note the areas where your body makes contact with the mattress. Breathe gently and deeply, letting yourself relax. Mentally list at least five things for which you are grateful, and install an inner and outer smile on your peaceful face. Take advantage of this tranquil moment!

Place your yoni egg on a part of your body that requires attention, or slide it beneath your pillow. If you own several different yoni eggs, choose one depending on your aspirations, your needs, and the properties of the stone from which it is made.

To proceed with programing an intention for the night, taking inspiration from Nicole Gratton, author of *L'art de rêver* [The art of dreaming], whom I had the pleasure of interviewing in Quebec, you might state: "Tonight, my intention is to remember my dreams and receive advice." Place your dream diary or personal journal next to your bed with a pencil so you are able to immediately write down every message that might arrive in the form of a dream over the course of the night, or when you wake up in the morning: "My dream has indicated to me that . . ."

❖ Ritual for a Couple

Suggesting to your partner that he or she practice a ritual with you will call for courage and openness, but the result will be magical, opening the gates of intimacy onto another dimension. In many tantric and Taoist traditions, the partners, for example, take a bath (what an ideal prelude) or a shower together, then clothe themselves in silk cloth, hold hands, look into each other's eyes, and express an intention for this moment. This gives them the means to enter a sacred space of kindness and creativity. This ritual will also have the intention of honoring your yoni as a couple.

After you have stated your intention, take your favorite yoni egg, present it to your partner, and suggest that he or she smear it with coconut oil and massage you with it. Your partner can then run it over the end of your mons veneris (pubic mound), over your labia, and over your clitoris before bringing it down toward your vagina and playing with it at the entrance. The stone egg might be cold at first contact, but this sensation could excite you (in the opposite case, do not hesitate to ask your partner to warm it up with his or her hands).

✛ Altar of Femininity

Choose a spot in your home for placing a symbol for the awakening of your femininity. This can be next to an image, a statue, or a painting or on a shelf on which you have arranged some personal objects that represent this stage. Make this a ritual space, defined and distinct from the other parts of your residence. In the best-case scenario, set it up in such a way that only you can have access to it. This is not so you can keep secrets but so that you can concentrate your energy, your intentions, your plans, and your harmony in this space for yourself. You can keep your egg here, and it will become imbued with all of the energy of this ritual space. In turn, it will give its own strength to this spot.

LOVE RITUALS FOR YOUR YONI

The rituals of the yoni will bring a great deal of love to this part of your body and pay it homage. The yoni is a sacred temple, the portal of your sacred feminine and of your creative energies. A little ritual is called for here, isn't it? This is a spot of your body that deserves to be celebrated, honored, revered, and adored. It is perfect just as it is, whatever its past, whatever its appearance or shape, and whatever its desires—and non-desires—may be.

Turn your attention toward the present and toward the future. Traumas, shame, guilt, and suffering, through your own personal history as well as that of your ancestors, steals from you a portion of your vitality, your creativity, and your inner wisdom. Through these rituals, you are going to make possible the beginning of a personal and meaningful relationship with this part of your body that has a lot to tell you.

✤ *Mirror, My Beautiful Mirror*

Take your most beautiful mirror and express the intention of becoming better acquainted with your yoni.

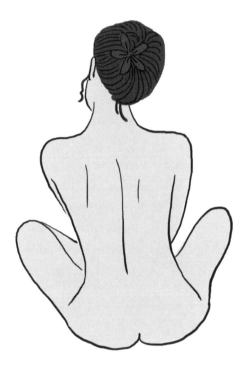

Figure 10.2. Gazing in the mirror

Use the mirror to observe your yoni for at least five minutes: its shape, its lips, its size, its texture, its color, and so forth. Every yoni is different, and there are so many women! Don't be tempted to judge at all. Love it as it is.

✤ *Message of the Yoni*

Choose a nice piece of paper or a small notebook that inspires you in which you can record the messages from your yoni. Decide how much time you are going to devote to this ritual and express the intention of writing down everything that your yoni has to tell you.

Light a candle, relax yourself into the present moment, and state your intention ("My intention is to release the memories of my yoni" or "My intention is to receive words of wisdom about my relationship"). Then start writing down what you hear and think without stopping, giving yourself permission to freely express everything that comes to you—everything that your yoni has to say to you. Do not judge what you are writing down. Just simply write it down. After you have learned what the message is, follow your intuition in deciding whether it would be best to free this text, destroy it, or anchor it. Perhaps you will choose to burn it, to decorate it, to keep it, to frame it, or to stick it in an album. Give free rein to your imagination and to your feminine creativity.

When you are done, give your thanks. Take action if some of the recommendations that you have received resonate in your heart.

❖ Yoni Massage

Bring organic coconut oil to a lukewarm temperature by running the container under hot water from the faucet. Dip your fingers into the oil and begin massaging your yoni—with lots of love and without any judgment, like a massage of unconditional love—into your belly and your yoni, both inside and out. Take your time; this is something nice you can do for yourself! Put an emphasis on each part of the yoni and surrounding area: urethra, vagina, anus, labia, clitoris, and so forth.

Perform this massage with presence, love, and awareness. Like you do for every ritual, light a candle, create an ambience, and express an intention of liberation, of contact with your sacred feminine and your inner wisdom.

❖ Celebration of Your Yoni

Choose a sculpture, a painting, a drawing, or an object that represents the yoni to you. The ritual itself can be undertaken in many different ways, but it is essential to include some elements with powerful symbolism. It is your job to discover what these elements are.

Begin the ritual with an act of reverence or a salutation before the representation of the yoni that you have chosen. Offer it flowers, fruits, rose petals, mantras, songs, or texts. These offerings should represent the five elements (earth, water, fire, spirit, air). Celebrate the yoni in your own personal way.

✦ New Moon or Full Moon Ritual

Grab your calendar! Note when the next full and new moons are occurring.

A new moon marks the beginning of a new cycle, which is an opportunity to open a new chapter of your life and to express intentions that inspire you. The full moon, on the other hand, is the time when feminine power is at its peak. Both, therefore, are ideal times for releasing the past, calling in the new, and using your yoni egg. There are countless ways to set up rituals around the new moon and the full moon. Here again, it is up to you to decide—candle, stone, yoni egg, music, or text—what will best represent for you the confidence you feel toward your creative prowess and the sacred feminine so as to manifest your most deeply personal intentions.

RITUALS FOR THE ENERGETIC CLEANSING OF YOUR YONI EGG

Yoni eggs are made of stone. They therefore originate in the earth and, consequently, contain the energy of life. Once they are no longer in contact with the earth, it is important to take care of them and maintain that energy. Before you use your egg for the first time, carefully clean your stone to rid it of the energies of other people who have touched it. Perhaps you already own several stones and have a regular practice? Carrying out an energy cleansing once or twice a month is a very good idea. Increase the frequency of these cleansings if you are going through a difficult time.

You can create your own cleansing rituals by simply following your intuition. Estelle, for example, gave free rein to her imagination.

❝ *I really love to perform rituals. To 'tame'
my egg, I invented one.*
ESTELLE **❞**

There are an infinite number of possibilities for energetically cleansing your egg. A ritual is a symbolic act. To carry one out, you will need a moment for yourself, alone, in a place that inspires you (at home or in nature). Begin with your intention—for example, "My intention is to practice a creative and spontaneous ritual that will allow me to energetically cleanse my yoni egg." You may be guided to use incense, sage, soft music, rose petals, gemstones, or prayers. The idea is to listen to your heart, your intention, and to let your intuition and soul guide you.

❝ *I clean the eggs after every time I use them,
and I put them in the sun for an entire day to
reenergize and purify them.*
CATHY **❞**

✤ At the Time of the Full Moon

Female energy is at its peak during the time of the full moon. Performing a cleansing ritual during this span of time is ideal, just as it is for using your yoni egg. Note the dates of the full moon in advance in your calendar. This will serve as a reminder of when to do an energy cleansing of your yoni egg.

❝ *I regularly place my yoni eggs in a beautiful
glass goblet and expose them for as long as possible
to the sun or, if it is at night, to the full moon.*
CAROLINE **❞**

On the evenings of the full moon, grant yourself a moment to take care of yourself. Take your egg with you if you like. Run a bath full of salted water or exfoliate your body. Light several candles and put on some soft and relaxing music, like the mantras of Deva Premal, which will encourage the awakening of the goddess within you—one who knows how to go about taking care of rituals and stones! Next, take a piece of silken cloth, place your egg on top of it, and set the cloth and egg in a place that will welcome them comfortably, like a sanctuary. Add flowers, candles, and incense, if you like. Practice your chosen form of meditation. That night, place your egg on your windowsill so that it can gorge on the light of the moon. Put it back in its sanctuary the next morning.

✤ Sage and Palo Santo

These shamanic methods are excellent for energetically cleansing a place, an individual, ourselves, a stone, or any other being, place, or object. But they will all be for naught without the formulation of intention for this energy cleansing.

So, begin by stating your intention, and then light a bundle of dried sage or a stick of palo santo (a Brazilian wood used for purification). Blow on the burning plant material to activate it. Then pass the burning herb in a circle around your yoni egg while asking Life and Source to sever all connections with any negative energy. Ask them to purify the egg. Take advantage of this opportunity to do the same to yourself and the room in which you find yourself. Listen to your intuition and let it be your guide. Liberate the goddess and the shaman who are within you.

✤ The Energy of Your Hands

If you are an energy worker, if you have healing powers, or if you practice Reiki or any other kind of energy medicine technique, it will be quite easy for you to energize your yoni egg with your hands. If you are unfamiliar with the experience of feeling energy travel through your hands, begin by vigorously rubbing them together, then separate them by a few scant inches and feel the energy they are releasing. Take your egg and direct the energy in your hands to travel through it. It is important to point out that passing the energy to the egg does not involve any mental activity; it is not you who is having any effect on your egg. You are simply allowing yourself to be penetrated by the energy of life, which is then infused quite naturally into your egg.

✤ Sound Vibrations

There are many vibrational instruments, such as Tibetan singing bowls, crystal bowls, and gongs, that make it possible to cause your gemstone egg to vibrate. It adores this, just as your body and its cells adore it. Take advantage of this time to state some beautiful intentions, and feel the benefit of each intention in every fiber of your being.

✤ With Water and Salt

Place your yoni egg in your sink and let water flow over it for several minutes. Visualize the egg and its energies being purified.

Immersion in saltwater is also recommended, but only for a short duration (less than fifteen minutes). It is also only advisable for certain stones, as salt can have a corrosive effect on some crystals.

If you live near the ocean, swim with your stone in the ocean's water, either holding the egg in your hand or keeping it tied to you with its string.

CREATING A WOMEN'S CIRCLE

We do not often take enough time to gather together with friends or just simply meet up with other women. However, these kinds of gatherings can do us so much good! Social networking, texts, and quick phone calls can never replace a meaningful and intimate moment together with friends.

Finding yourself in the company of other conscious and living women is powerful. There are numerous opportunities to bring women together: a birth, the new moon, the yoni egg practice, the opening of a new chapter of life, and so forth.

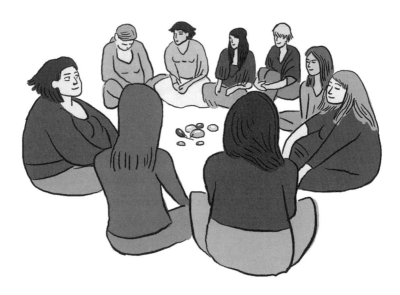

Figure 10.3. Women's circle

A women's circle makes it possible to create a network of energetic support for the women present. At the same time, it makes that energetic support available for all the women in the world. It makes a return into sacred space possible.

Priestess Suzanne Sterling confirms: "Our frequencies synchronize when we are together in a group. When we sing, dance, and pray together, our minds shut down."

As is the case with any ritual, the idea is to let yourself give free rein to your imagination and your creativity by allowing yourself to be guided by what you do well. Have fun, laugh, honor the goddess that is you, read inspiring writings, share, and fully experience the present moment.

Ask each of the women invited to be part of this circle to bring their favorite essential oil, their favorite stones or crystals, and, if they own them, their yoni eggs, as well as some flowers, rose petals, or herbs.

Prepare the place where you will be gathering so that it is beautiful and filled with an atmosphere of gentleness and kindness. Place cloth drapes and hangings over the floor (red is a good color because it is evocative of menstrual blood), scatter cushions, and fill the room with flowers.

Purify all the women who come with the help of sage or palo santo. Then all the women should join hands and form a circle together. Every person there will share her intention with the rest of this circle of women.

Sing, read poems, meditate, and dance. Immerse yourself in a feeling of joy and the sharing of the present moment, connected to your family tree and all the women in the world. If you like, use a talking stick to make sure that everyone there is able to speak in turn.

The yoni egg will also have its place in this women's circle. Use the circle as an opportunity to pass on information about the egg to other women who may not yet have had an opportunity to know the yoni egg and experience its revelatory and liberating effects on female power.

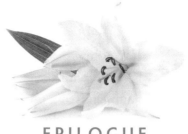

A Delightful Adventure

What a wonderful time to be a woman living on Earth! We are experiencing a paradigm shift in which the feminine principle is reawakening in all its splendor. It is such a joy to have the opportunity to be a witness and actress in this momentous change, isn't it?

I really want you—individually or collectively—to be able to take advantage of all the moments that are offered to you to create your life day after day with beauty and creativity. May they give you the desire to explore, to free yourself, and to enjoy every opportunity that majestically presents itself to you.

The yoni egg can accompany you in these different phases of life and in the opening of this new chapter. Freeing our inner wisdom and inner beauty is something that is possible to all of us. There has never been a better time than now. Of course, the yoni egg is not the only tool you can use to do this, but it is, in my opinion, a gateway to access more of who you are, the part that hasn't been liberated and expressing itself yet. The fact that the use of the yoni egg has never been more widely known than it is today, that it has been revealed to countless women in all four corners of the world, shows that the time has come to be radiant and rediscover the path of the sacred feminine. You are a goddess. You are guided.

May delightful discoveries and adventures come to all of you.

With all my heart,
Lilou Macé

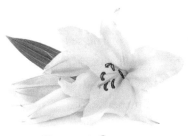

Postface

By Aisha Sieburth

There it is; you now have had a taste of the first stages of the yoni egg practice, and you are feeling unprecedented effects that are already inviting you to explore more deeply the hidden treasures of your secret sources. Welcome to the journey of discovery of your sacred feminine!

The practice of the yoni egg has been designed to awaken the sacred dimension of female energy so that women will have the ability to reconnect to its gentleness, its healing energy, and its tranquil strength. By exercising regularly with the internal movements of the yoni egg, you will succeed in awakening your deep energy. You will cultivate the inner power of the orgasmic frequency that will become a complete tool for self-healing when dealing with common disorders. For men, the awakening of sacred masculine energy will be achieved through specific practices of cultivation and mastery designed to tame their energy and develop their sexual potency.

Once the individual training has been successfully achieved, then the natural merger of yin and yang can be developed within the intimate confines of the couple. This union of forces will augment the love energy that is present and direct it toward what is called the "multi-orgasm." This multi-orgasm has such powerful creative energy that it illuminates the body, heart, and spirit. Sexual energy, transmuted into a vital force in the couple's life, opens a window on to the fabled horizons of the reconciliation of the sexes and their complementarity.

Mastery of this formidable energy requires times and working to anchor it in your very bedrock so that the energy can circulate properly in your body. This is an immense program that demands patience, complicity, and, most importantly, love. Sexuality will then make itself the starting point for the formidable adventure of life.

Good practice! And good chi to you!

AISHA SIEBURTH is a senior instructor of the Universal Healing Tao System and the coauthor with Master Mantak Chia of *Chi Nei Tsang and Microcurrent Therapy* and *Life Pulse Massage*. She lives and works in Avignon, France, as director of the School of the Tao of Vitality and Soulimet Association.

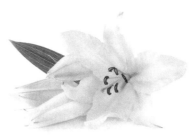

Resources and More about the Author

Lilou Macé, author and interviewer, is the creator of numerous interviews, video blogs, books, websites, and events. She has been recognized as an international reference on the internet since 2006, with more than one hundred million views on YouTube.

Lilou has been traveling across the world since 2011 to interview authors, therapists, scientists, and celebrities in search of a more global, inspiring understanding of our lives. Beyond cultures, dogmas, and countries, Lilou brings together the visible and the invisible, the material and the spiritual, the rational and the intuitive. She shows that unification is not only possible but also necessary for our evolution and for our society.

You can find her books, cards, and more at liloumace.com/en/my -store. Here you can also find a beautiful selection of yoni eggs.

CONTACTING THE AUTHOR

I welcome all your testimonies and questions. Share with me what the yoni egg has revealed about you as well as what your favorite practices and rituals are, including those you have created yourself, and your advice for other women. Contact me at **lateledelilou@gmail.com** or

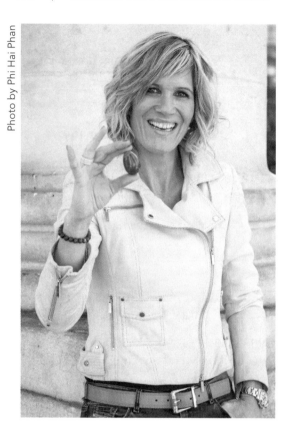

Photo by Phi Hai Phan

visit me online at **www.liloumace.com/en**, where I post my agenda, new videos, and other materials in English.

OTHER USEFUL ONLINE RESOURCES

Mantak Chia: http://www.mantakchia.com
Jutta Kellenberger: http://www.juttakellenberger.com
Aisha Sieburth: http://www.taodelavitalite.org
Minke de Vos: http://www.femininetreasures.com/minke
Solla Pizzuto: http://www.sourcetantra.com
Shashi Solluna: http://shashisolluna.com
Saida Desilets: http://www.SaidaDesilets.com

INTERVIEWS THAT CONTRIBUTED TO THE WRITING OF THIS BOOK

These interviews are primarily in English and available on YouTube by typing the title of the interview into the search bar. Note that these titles are recorded here to match the exact titles on You Tube, inclusive of errors, so that they can be found easily.

Interviews with Mantak Chia

"Mantak Chia: Tao's Sexual and Multi-Orgasmic Practices for Longevity – Part 1"

"Darkroom's Organic Visions Vs. Magic Mushrooms and Drugs – Mantak Chia part 2"

"Part 1/5 – How to Have a Brain Orgasm and Why? Mantak Chia"

"Part 2/5 – Prevent Prostate Caner with Prostate Gland Massage in Anus Near G Spot – Mantak Chia"

"Part 3/5 – Healing of the Female Ejaculation – Mantak Chia"

"Part 4/5 – Death Hormone, Ayahuasca and Kidney Energy – Mantak Chia"

"Jade Egg Practices – Mantak Chia Part 5"

Interviews with Sarina Stone

"Sexual Energy, Energizing Organs and Seminal Retention for Longevity – Sarina Stone"

"Comment libérer son chi et énergie sexuelle? Sarina Stone" (in French)

Interviews with Aisha Sieburth

"Life Pulse Massage and Sexual Energy – Tao with Aisha Sieburth"

"Qu'est ce que le Tao? Comment se guérir grâce à votre énergie sexuelle? – Aisha Sieburth" (in French)

"Pratiques de l'oeuf de jade (l'oeuf de yoni) – Aisha Sieburth" (in French)

Interviews with José Toirán

"How to Control My Ejaculation? José Toirán (Part 3)"

"(VF) Comment atteindre un plus grand orgasme (homme & femme)" (in French)

"Énergie sexuelle, orgasmes et oeuf de jade – José Toiràn" (in French)

Interview with Jutta Kellenberger
"Practice of the Jade Egg for Sacred Feminine – Jutta Kellenberger"

Interview with Minke de Vos
"Sacred Femininity and Jade Egg Practices – Minke de Vos"

Interview with Shashi Solluna
"How Sexual Penetration Impact Our Energy as Women – Shashi Solluna"

Interview with Solla Pizzuto
"The Jade Egg Practices – Solla Pizzuto Part2"

OTHER CONTRIBUTORS TO THIS BOOK

Corinne Léger
Corinne, an osteopath in Margaux in the Gironde region (Bordeaux), has been practicing osteopathy since 1994. She is passionate about energy healing treatments like stone therapy, essential oils, sound therapy, and emotional homeopathy.

Elizabeth Beaumont
Elizabeth is a gemologist with a degree from the the Gemmological Association of Great Britain (Gem-A). She is also a certified appraiser of the School of Gemmology in Montreal, whose courses are certified by the Canadian Jewelers Association Accredited Appraiser Program and also by Gemworld International.

François Lehn
François has been a science/health journalist, specializing in new approaches to health and complementary care, for more than fifteen years. His website, Presse Santé, features information and news about natural health topics.

Index